Departing
with Dignity

A hospice guide to symptom management
for PATIENTS, FAMILIES and CAREGIVERS

WILLIAM R. NESBITT, III, M.D.
WITH JAMES McGREGOR, M.D.

ISBN-13: 9780578483252

Edited and Typeset by Amnet Systems.
Cover design by Amnet Systems.

DEDICATION

To all the forward-thinking, dedicated medical professionals, administrators, organizations, and public servants who are contributing to the transformation of medical care by the promotion of hospice and palliative medicine.

And most importantly, this book is also dedicated to all the courageous hospice staff, families, friends, and caregivers who selflessly attend to those experiencing the very end of their journey here on earth.

To all these individuals, we give our most profound admiration and thanks.

CONTENTS

Introduction: About Us   vii

1   What Is Hospice?   1
2   Is It Time for Hospice?   14
3   Charting Your Course with Advance Directives   23
4   Managing Pain   33
5   Managing Constipation and Diarrhea   47
6   Managing Shortness of Breath   54
7   Managing Agitation and Delirium   60
8   Preventing Falls   65
9   Managing Nausea and Vomiting   72
10 Management and Prevention of Skin Breakdown   79
11 Managing Sleep   85
12 Managing Bleeding   91
13 Medications   97
14 Tube Feeding   104
15 Knowing the End Is Near   113
16 Final Thoughts   123

INTRODUCTION:
ABOUT US

Jim and I decided to write this book because of the enormous and growing need for help with end-of-life care. Also, we have grown aware of the need to help change the culture in this country regarding attitudes toward life's completion in this physical world in which our bodies exist. But in our modern Western culture, we do not speak of the end of life, let alone integrate it into our daily lives. Although we know in our *heads* that we are mortal, we usually do not realize this in our *hearts* until we are faced with the impending and inevitable reality of death. Because the end of life is something everyone will experience, we are endeavoring to create a resource for patients, families, and caregivers to help with home symptom management and to help you know what to say to guide your doctor in the right direction in addressing questions over the phone.

Our journeys into this field of medicine began early in our lives. Our personal confrontations with the death of loved ones in our early years were our first steps leading us ultimately to careers in hospice and palliative medicine.

Jim was raised on a small farm in Ontario, Canada. His heart was first broken as a young child when death took his beloved old dog, who passed peacefully in the warm grass of a beautiful green hill. More unfair was when his pet lamb Blackie had his life cut short by eating poisonous plants.

But nothing could have prepared him, at age twenty, for the horrible tragedy of losing both his parents in a motor vehicle accident. As he tried to sleep upstairs in his room, he was surprised at the lack of community support there was for him and his sisters as he endured the emptiness and sorrow, with his parents' caskets downstairs in the living room after a day of visitation at the farmhouse.

Determined that this bleak experience should not be endured by others, in 1981 he helped establish the first palliative care team at a regional hospital in Ontario. Since then he has worked tirelessly to help develop hospice and palliative medicine programs in Ontario and then since 1997, in Northern California. Jim became a national figure in end-of-life care when he demonstrated how the palliative care program he helped develop saved the health care system millions of dollars and improved the quality of the time those patients had left.

As a child, my first encounter with death was when my four-year-old playmate died of meningitis. My father, a doctor, comforted us children and helped us to understand that life was unpredictable and death could come unexpectedly for anyone. His compassion and care comforted us greatly, and since that time I knew I wanted to be a physician like him. Because of my many long talks with my father regarding life, death, and spiritual things, I was better prepared for the tragedy I experienced at age sixteen. On a mountain trail one night, a friend of mine slipped and fell off a thirty-foot cliff into a creek, right before my eyes. I tried to climb down the cliff to save him, but I ended up falling as well. I was able to find him and pulled him from the icy water. It was only when rescuers came that I found out he had died and I had broken my arm. Tragedy visited again when I came home from college to hear that my best friend growing up had committed suicide.

I went on to medical school after receiving my undergraduate degree in psychology. After my family-practice residency and five years working as an emergency-department physician, I went into family medicine. That is when I met Jim in1997. As he was assisting in developing our community's hospice program, I took over care of the bulk of the area's nursing-home patients and care homes for the developmentally disabled. During this time my passion for hospice care grew as I saw the great need in the facilities I served. Both Jim and I received our advanced certifications in hospice and palliative medicine as well as Hospice Medical Director certification. I joined Jim's hospice team with Sutter Health in 2013, and we have been working together ever since.

At this time, we are leaving clinical practice and are changing course in our careers in order to teach others the many lessons we have learned in our years in hospice. This book is just a start. Every one of us is going to face death, and every physician is going to deal with dying patients and their families. Although this book is targeted at patients and their families and caregivers, the information that we share is essential for professional clinicians as well in providing excellent care to patients.

And finally, we wish to share some of the hospice experiences we have had that may give us a peek behind death's dark curtain. These amazing experiences may indicate that death of the body is not the end of our conscious lives. Every hospice has stories like these. We include these stories to give hope in such dark times. We simply state these stories as they were told to us by hospice staff and families. The interpretation of these accounts, as well as their implications regarding the meaning of life, spiritual realities that exist as certainly as physical realities, and what this may mean for how we live our lives, this is all beyond the scope of this book (but maybe not our next one).

In addition to providing comfort and dignity in the last days of those we love, we hope that the information that follows will give patients, families, and caregivers some of the comfort, hope, and meaning that we have received during our many years of caring for those on the brink of eternity.

1

WHAT IS HOSPICE?

As a patient progresses through a chronic illness, such as heart failure, Alzheimer's disease, or emphysema, usual medical treatment will aggressively manage the disease with the primary goal of extending life. Patients and families may be under the misconception that the patient is going to get better, as one does from a sore throat or a broken arm. Early in the disease process, it is rare for physicians to begin discussions regarding how the disease will affect the quality and length of their patients' lives as the disease progresses. Frank and detailed discussions are uncommon about when and how the goals of treatment should change over time. Physicians do not want to give patients "bad news." They justify avoiding these discussions by saying they do not want to take away the patient's hope. Unfortunately, for all human beings, most chronic illnesses will ultimately be a losing battle. Our ancient enemy, Death, will claim us all in the end.

When a doctor practices usual medical care, it is easy to be blinded to the inevitability of death, given all the marvelous advancements in health care as well as the abundant treatment options available. In a perfect world, physicians would begin preparing their patients early in the game when they are diagnosed with a condition that cannot be cured but only managed. Issues such as advance directives and durable power of attorney for health care should be brought up. A smooth transition should occur with an increasing focus on symptom management and a decreasing focus on unrealistic attempts at life prolongation. The transition from usual medical care to hospice care is known as "palliative care." This is where the focus on easing symptoms, rather than curing the disease, occurs. Palliative care should begin when the patient is likely to have a life expectancy of two to five years.

A major problem, however, is that physicians are notoriously bad at estimating prognosis, or how long a patient is likely to live. I cannot recall a single lecture in medical school regarding prognosis. It is so bad that on the Hospice and Palliative Medicine Board Exam, for the question, "By how much on average do physicians overestimate how long a patient will live?" the correct answer is "By a factor of three." That means if the doctor says grandma has six months to live, she is not likely to be around eight to ten weeks later. Patients are generally referred to hospice way too late in the disease because of the doctor's poor prognostic skills or the doctor not wanting to "just give up."

The doctor may not want the patient to lose hope (even when the condition is hopeless). In hospice, false hope may be replaced with real hope. Restoration and reconciliation of relationships in this life, reduction in suffering, a peaceful and dignified passing, and reuniting with the loved ones who have gone before you, become realistic hopes and achievable goals through hospice. Evidence that these goals can be achieved will be discussed in later chapters. Also, the patient may not be aware of how limited their time is. As tricky as prognosis might be, given the dozens of factors that need to be considered, there are some pretty good guidelines that can be helpful in knowing when it is time for hospice. These will be discussed in a later chapter.

Another reason hospice is underutilized or delayed is the set of myths about it. For example, "It is a betrayal of my loved one not to keep fighting" or "Hospice is for patients in their last hours or days of life" or "On hospice they stop everything and just put you on morphine and oxygen." The truth is recognizing that continuing futile aggressive care increases and prolongs suffering and earlier hospice intervention results in better symptom control and often longer survival than with usual medical care.

Eligibility for hospice is achieved when two physicians determine a patient's life expectancy is for six months or less if the illness runs its usual course. Usually, patients are referred by their physicians, who attest to their six-months-or-less prognosis, and a second confirmation of prognosis is made by the hospice medical director. When patients or families reach out on their own to hospice because they do not have a regular doctor in the area, the hospice medical director can act as the attending physician. Many primary care doctors prefer the Hospice Medical Director assume the patient's care, but it is always the patient's choice as to who will be the attending physician. Often patients are referred to hospice while in the hospital by the hospital physician, and patients and families may decide who manages their care from there.

Once referred, the patients are interviewed by members of the hospice team to confirm eligibility and then to help them determine their goals of care. Hospice patients are ones who have arrived at the point where they wish to be kept comfortable at home rather than continue to attack their disease, which often comes at a high cost to their quality (and sometimes even the quantity) of their life. Most of the time a patient has the sense that he or she is dying, often before even the physician is willing to admit it. These patients find that they would rather reprioritize their lives and prefer to live out the rest of their lives in comfort at home with their families rather than going back and forth to the hospital, consuming their precious last days with futile treatments and unnecessary tests.

For those patients on Medicare (as most hospice eligible patients are), there is no cost to the patient for hospice care. Other covered benefits are medications related to the terminal illness. Medications for concurrent serious illnesses contributing to the patient's decline are covered as well. Any tests, treatments, therapies, or specialty referrals needed for management of the patient's terminal symptoms may also be covered. In addition, artificial nutrition or hydration, or external respiration assistance, that will reduce symptoms, increase self-care function, or decrease caregiver burden will also usually be covered by hospice. Therapies simply for rehabilitation, or aggressive measures, treatments, or therapies to prevent potential symptoms or merely for life prolongation, are not covered benefits. Therapies and medications unrelated to the terminal diagnosis would continue to be paid for by Medicare or the patient's insurance. Many non-Medicare insurances offer a hospice benefit similar to Medicare.

When the patient chooses to enter hospice, his or her care is managed by the hospice interdisciplinary team (IDT), which consists of a nurse, a physician, a social worker, a chaplain, and a home health aide. The patient's primary physician may direct the care or, as is more often the case, their physician will turn over the care to the hospice medical director, who is usually more skilled and qualified at dealing with difficult issues of end-of-life medical management. The goal is to help the family or other caregivers to learn to provide end-of-life care for the patient at home or in any facility where the patient resides.

The case manager nurse is the primary point of contact with the patient and family and visits as often as needed, from multiple times a day during crisis situations, to once every week or two if the patient is very stable. He or she does most of the assessments, care, education, medication organization, and communication with the medical director or hospice team physician. The physician gives orders based on the nurse's recommendations, visits the home, if necessary, for severe-symptom management or recertification or discharge visits. He or she also reviews the patient's condition, plan of care, and medications in the weekly meetings and provides the extensive documentation for Medicare or other insurance.

Social workers assess the safety, stability, and appropriateness of the patients' living arrangements and support structure and assist the family in final arrangements with mortuaries. Social workers may assist in accessing community resources and help with paperwork such as FMLA, utility discounts, proof of hospice services, provide psychological support for the family, and too many other services to mention. The chaplain helps the patient and the family with religious and existential concerns, assists in finding visiting clergy of the patient's choosing, and supports the patient with prayer, songs, counseling, or just active listening as the patient wishes. The home health aides help with bathing, personal care, companionship, reading, or sitting with the patient while a family member runs an errand.

There are four levels of hospice care: routine home care, continuous care, general inpatient care, and respite care. Should symptoms such as pain, shortness of breath, vomiting, or agitation require prolonged direct supervision by the nurse, the patient can be put on "continuous care" status until symptoms are again manageable by the family or facility. If symptoms are too severe to be managed at home, the patient can be put on "general inpatient" (GIP) status either in the hospital or a qualified skilled nursing facility, where medications can be rapidly adjusted under close medical supervision and yet remain under the care of the hospice team.

"General inpatient" status cannot be chosen as a final destination. It is for temporary management of symptoms only. For Medicare to pay under GIP status, a discharge plan must be in place or be developing. If, however, the patient dies during symptom control, or while developing a plan of care that can be duplicated at home or another facility, Medicare will cover the GIP hospice stay. If the family needs a break either due to being overwhelmed by care-giving or a need to attend to urgent matters out of town, the patient may be admitted to a skilled nursing facility or RCFE for up to five days under "respite care." There are no strict Medicare guidelines for how often respite care can be used. However, clear documentation is needed to justify the hospice respite-care status. Long-term custodial care is not covered under the hospice benefit.

Medicare pays the hospice organization a daily rate, based on the levels of care as mentioned above, for all care and medications related to the patient's terminal condition. Medicaid and many private insurances make similar arrangements with the hospice. Again, the Medicare hospice benefit does not pay for nursing home stays for hospice patients except for the days the patient is at a skilled nursing facility on "general inpatient status" or "respite status." However, Medicaid can cover long-term nursing home stays if the patient qualifies under Medicaid financial guidelines.

When a patient first enrolls in hospice, they are certified for ninety days. If the patient survives this ninety-day period, they can be recertified for a second ninety-day period without a face-to-face physician or nurse practitioner examination, as long as they still meet criteria for a six-month-or-less prognosis. If the patient survives the second ninety-day benefit period, either the hospice team physician, the medical director, or the hospice nurse practitioner must visit the patient to confirm their six-month-or-less prognosis. If the patient still qualifies, they will be recertified for sixty-day periods, which requires a physician or nurse practitioner's face-to-face visit each time. If at any time the patient appears to have stabilized or improved to the point where it is likely they will live longer than six months, the patient will be discharged back to their physician until such a time as their condition again begins to decline. Very frequently we see patients who, prior to hospice, were in and out of the hospital every couple of weeks. However, on hospice, with better symptom and medication management, we often see those patients go for months remaining comfortable at home. An additional benefit of hospice is bereavement support services to the family for thirteen months after the patient passes.

Patients can revoke hospice services at any time and for any reason, such as wishing to pursue aggressive/curative care again. In addition, patients who revoke hospice or are discharged may re-enroll at any time as long as they still qualify under the six-month prognosis guideline. Patients can be discharged from hospice if their condition (and therefore their prognosis) improves. If the family disagrees with the decision to discharge, there is an appeal process that they can access. There is much more about the financial and regulatory aspects of hospice, beyond the scope of this book, which can be obtained on the Internet or from a local hospice organization.

Under hospice, comfort and quality of life replace function and cure as the primary goals. When pain management interferes with function, the team tries as much as possible to let the patient determine the desired balance between alertness and sedation. Patients will often be willing to put up with quite a bit of pain at times in order to enjoy their family as long as they can. Working with the patient's primary physician, the patient's medication regimen is simplified as much as possible. Preventive medications such as cholesterol meds, blood thinners, and vitamins and supplements are usually discontinued, as they can cause side effects; drug interactions can increase the burden of taking pills, as it becomes more difficult to swallow. More on medications in a later chapter.

As the patient's general condition deteriorates, all medications except comfort medications are discontinued. Hospice comfort medications are formulated so that in most cases they can still be administered without IVs or injections even to the patients who can no longer swallow or are no longer conscious. Ironically, some patients improve dramatically once all their medications have been stopped. It is frequently the case that side-effects and interactions of medications were actually responsible for their decline. We had one elderly lady who came to us not eating or drinking, no longer able to walk, only able to mumble a few words, and no longer able to care for herself. When we stopped twenty-four of her twenty-six medications, she began walking, talking, and eating again and was discharged due to extended prognosis.

The greatest mistake is waiting too long to enroll in hospice services. Too often doctors wait till it's way too late in the process to refer a patient to hospice care. We sometimes receive referrals only minutes before the patient expires. The earlier we can get patients in the six-month window, the sooner we can maximize symptom control and quality of life. There are usually two stages for our hospice patients. Early in the course, we prioritize function as well as symptom management. For example, life sustaining measures such as cardiac and respiratory medications are continued and optimized. In certain cases, dialysis patients can continue their treatments if they have been stable and the hospice diagnosis is something unrelated, like a brain tumor. We want our patients to get the most comfort out of their time remaining. When the disease progresses and the patient transitions to the "actively dying stage," then function takes a back seat to comfort. Anything that may prolong the active dying process is stopped. Although symptoms can be very severe as the body struggles in resisting death, through appropriate management of medications and other modalities, we can control almost any suffering. The greatest challenge to symptom management is when patients are referred too late, as we sometimes need more time to dial in symptom control.

Hospice philosophy is guided by the four pillars of medical ethics: autonomy (honoring the patient's wishes), beneficence (doing what is good, right, and beneficial), nonmaleficence (doing no harm), and justice (i.e., what is fair to everyone). The principle of autonomy tells us that each patient should have the right, as much as possible, to be free to make informed decisions regarding their health care, and determine what they will and will not allow. When patients become unable or unwilling to express their own wishes, a decision maker of their choosing needs to be appointed to act on their behalf, to set the limits and seek to achieve the goals that the *patient* would want if the patient were able to make an informed decision themselves. It should be made clear that the decisions should not be based on the surrogate decision maker's personal values or wishes but on what the patient would want for themselves.

Beneficence means the team is committed to doing what is good, right, and helpful for the patient. This does not mean that aggressive curative treatments must always be pursued. The transition into this life, birth, is a natural process that proceeds at its own time and rate as long as all goes well. Dying, like birth, is also a natural process, an inevitable one for all who are born. The body works best at its natural pace. Just as we would not try to stop or prolong labor at the due date, prolonging the natural dying process can be as harmful to the patient as well. When it is impossible to prolong someone's *living*, it is wrong to prolong their *dying*, as it can greatly increase the severity and duration of suffering. Instead, utilizing the principle of honoring the wisdom of the body, we refrain from aggressive intrusions that disrupt the natural course of the body shutting down at its appointed time. We simply maintain the comfort and dignity of the individual as they prepare for their final departure.

Non-maleficence means that we do nothing to prevent the body from going through its inevitable, natural process of shutting down. But occasionally patients or their families will "just want it to be over" and request something to "speed things up." However, we cannot deliberately take an innocent life. If the patient is in pain, having difficulty breathing, intractable vomiting, seizures, or lingering for days in a coma, it would seem like the compassionate thing to do is to put them out of their misery. These situations can be very distressing to everyone including the hospice team. Fortunately, if the patient's suffering is the only thing keeping him alive, much can be done to stop the suffering and allow the body to naturally shut down as quickly as possible.

Justice means fairness, not only to an individual patient but also fairness to all who seek hospice care as well as for the society at large. All hospice patients should have equal access to all hospice resources without discrimination based on race, gender, religion, nationality, economic status, or political belief. In addition, the precious and limited resources of hospice must be managed by a sense of stewardship that does not allow resources to be wasted, when such use would be harmful or medically ineffective for the patient.

In summary, hospice is a caring multidisciplinary team of highly educated professionals who educate and teach the team of the family and their caregivers to care for their loved one in their last days at home. The time for hospice is when the patient has six months or less to live and wants to focus more on making each day the best that it can be, rather than wasting their precious remaining time simply trying to prolong the dying process. Costs to the patient are minimal, if any, and the benefits and services to the patient and family are abundant. The greatest mistake a patient or family can make at the end of life is not contacting hospice soon enough or at all.

2

IS IT TIME FOR HOSPICE?

Now that you know what hospice is, are you (or the loved one you are caring for) ready for hospice? If you have just been informed by your physician that it is time for hospice, the time is likely to be long overdue. As I mentioned previously, not only are we physicians reluctant to inform our patients of bad news, we are often very poorly trained in knowing when the bad news is staring us in the face. For years, I know this was true for me. In this chapter we will discuss how to let your physician know that you are not only willing to hear "bad news" but in dire need of that knowledge.

Most physicians are very compassionate people who often develop strong emotional bonds with their patients. This contributes to the fact that most physicians are overly optimistic of their patients' time left, do not want their patients to lose hope, and often have the false belief that patients do not want to know their prognosis (the time left). Considering this, asking, "So, Doc, how much time have I got?" may not give you the most useful information. Despite the fact that physicians usually grossly overestimate the patient's survival time, there are ways to get more of the information that you need.

To be fair to physicians, it must be said that no two patients are the same in terms of their mortality risk factors. Dozens of factors come into play. Concurrent chronic illnesses and their severity, concurrent acute illnesses and their severity, age, genetics, general physical fitness (not considering the terminal illness), adequacy of medical management of current problems, compliance with optimal treatment, potential side-effects and drug interactions, medication errors, falls and their injuries, depression, the will to live, recent death of a spouse, and cultural expectations are but a few of the confounding factors in predicting how long someone may live. Sometimes there is no way to predict survival time. Some of our patients with neurological decline could die tonight or a year or two from now. So where do we start?

In hospice we are taught the Buckman Protocol, which is a format for delivering bad news to patients. By modifying the protocol's questions a bit, the protocol can be used by the family or patient on the physician to elicit from your doctor information that you may not otherwise get. If you are concerned about whether or not it is time for Grandma to go on hospice, first, set up an appointment, an extended one (at least a half hour), "to review the patients overall health and discuss recommendations for the future plan of care." This should alert the physician of the patient and family's willingness and readiness to talk about tough issues.

At the appointment, when the physician asks what specifically you would like to talk about, start with, "I would like to first explain to you everything I understand about Grandma's condition, and then I would like you to fill me in on whatever I am leaving out." After describing your understanding of each of her diagnoses and the individual and combined impacts that they may have on her in the future, ask if you are unaware of any other conditions that may affect the quantity or quality of her life. Next, go over every medication that she is prescribed as well as the over-the-counter ones, including vitamins and supplements. Ask if there are any that should or could be reduced, discontinued, avoided, or may be causing side effects or drug interactions. (Much more on medications in a later chapter.)

Next, describe to the physician Grandma's current condition and changes (especially the declines) over the past few months. Things to include are weight changes, oral intake, ability to care for herself, bowel and bladder control, sleep pattern and amount, mental functioning, falls, mood swings, increase in assistance with self-care, any coughing with meals or difficulty swallowing, and any other concerns you may have. Finally, ask the "surprised" questions: "If you would be surprised to hear that she died tonight, how long before it would *not* surprise you to hear she had died?" and "How long before it would surprise you to hear she was still alive?" These questions may aid you in assessing how much time the patient really has. If the physician feels, based on your discussion, that Grandma is not likely to make it six months based on her diagnosis and/or rate of decline, she may well be eligible for hospice.

Besides the patient's rate of decline, there are also disease-specific criteria which, if present, put the patient at the statistical risk of death within six months. Even if these criteria are not met, if the rate of the patient's decline is steep enough that a six-month survival is unlikely, the patient still qualifies for hospice even if she doesn't meet criteria. I will include a few of the major illnesses and their indications that a six-month survival is unlikely. Here is a summary of some of the criteria in the great hospice handbook, *Hospice Quickflips*.

For **neurodegenerative disorders** like ALS (Lou Gehrig's Disease) or MS (multiple sclerosis), we look for increasing difficulty breathing at rest, rapid respiratory rate (more than 20 breaths per minute), weakened speech and cough, irregular breathing during sleep, increased time sleeping, or weight loss of 5 percent or more.

For **cancer,** it is a bad sign if the disease has spread to other parts of the body (Stage IV) at the time of diagnosis. Likewise, if the disease is spreading despite aggressive treatment, or if the patient is refusing treatment with stage IV disease, prognosis is likely to be less than six months. The most dangerous cancers, such as small-cell lung cancer, brain cancer, or pancreatic cancer, may qualify for hospice earlier than stage IV.

With **coma,** if the brainstem is affected, if the patient is not able to speak or does not respond to pain, prognosis is poor enough for hospice. Factors confirming a grim prognosis include urinary infections, pneumonia from difficulty swallowing, fevers that don't respond to antibiotics, and deep nonhealing wounds from skin breakdown. Prognosis worsens with larger strokes with either bleeding or blood-vessel blockages.

For **dementia from Alzheimer's disease** (not the kind related to multiple small strokes), the loss of ability to walk, dress, or bathe, loss of bowel and bladder control, or reduction in speech to six words or less, are bad signs. Other factors include the patient having urinary infections in the past few months that have spread to the blood stream, lung infections from difficulty swallowing, blood infections, multiple deep pressure sores, or recurring fevers after antibiotics. To this list you can add dehydration, inability to take in adequate nutrition with a 10 percent weight loss in the past six months, and/or low protein blood levels.

For admission to hospice based on the eligibility criteria below, a patient with **heart disease** must have optimum medical management of their illness. The patient must not be a candidate for corrective procedures or refuse optimal or corrective care. The patient with heart failure or coronary artery disease qualifies for hospice if they have symptoms at rest and cannot engage in any physical activity, and/or the heart's output is very poor (less than 20 percent). Treatment-resistant irregular heart rhythms, history of cardiac arrest, unexplained fainting, strokes from blood clots in the heart, and/or concurrent HIV disease are additional risk factors.

In **HIV disease**, hospice-qualifying factors are quite technical, and include 10 percent or more loss of lean body mass, low CD4+ count (greater than 25 cells/mcl), certain cancers (unresponsive visceral Kaposi sarcoma, CNS lymphoma, systemic lymphoma), certain infections (unresponsive or untreated MAC (mycobacterium avium complex), cryptosporidium, unresponsive toxoplasmosis), kidney failure, PML (progressive multifocal leukoencephalopathy), along with a decline in function to the point that the patient is mostly sitting or lying, unable to do any work, requires considerable assistance with self-care, may have reduced intake, and may become confused. Additional risk factors include being over fifty years of age, active substance abuse, more than a year of chronic diarrhea, or advanced AIDS dementia complex.

Liver disease qualifies with the combination of certain lab tests (INR greater than 1.5 and albumen less than 2.5) plus signs of end-stage liver disease such as ascites (abdominal cavity fluid), infection of that fluid, concurrent kidney failure, resistant or untreatable confusion, lethargy or coma due to liver disease, or recurrent bleeding from varicose veins in the esophagus. Prognosis is worse with liver cancer, Hepatitis B or C, continued active alcoholism, progressive malnutrition, or increasing weakness requiring increasing help with self-care.

Lung disease qualifies with disabling shortness of breath at rest despite inhaled medications, confinement to bed or chair, increasing emergency room visits and hospital admissions, low blood oxygen (less than 88 percent on room air), or increased CO2 in the blood (pCO2 greater than 50mmHg). Right-sided heart failure, weight loss, and resting rapid heart rate (less than 100/minute) all increase risk as well.

Kidney failure qualifies if the patient is not a candidate for dialysis, or declines dialysis or renal transplantation, has very low kidney function (CrCl<10cc/min—in diabetics or heart failure patients, creatinine>8—over 6 in diabetics, eGFR<10ml/min). Other serious concurrent illnesses worsen prognosis as well.

Stroke qualifies if the patient is mainly bedbound, unable to do most activities, requires almost total care, has markedly reduced intake of food and liquids and is not obtaining those essential requirements from tube feeding or IVs, and normal or reduced level of consciousness, with or without confusion. In addition, the patient must be unable to maintain adequate nutrition and hydration as noted by a weight loss of 10 percent in the past six months or 7.5 percent in the past three months. The patient also must have worsening difficulty swallowing preventing adequate intake (without artificial nutrition) and resulting in lung infections.

Regardless of the specific disease under which the patient was admitted, there are several indicators to show if that the condition is worsening or the rate of decline is steepening. A partial list includes the following: recurring infections, less than 10 percent weight loss in the past six months, increased trouble swallowing, declining levels of albumin or cholesterol, declining levels of white or red blood cell (leukopenia or anemia) without another known cause, worsening shortness of breath, intractable nausea, vomiting or diarrhea, worsening pain requiring increasing doses of medication, dropping blood pressure, development of blood clots or edema, declining strength or function, decline in mental functioning, worsening deep skin break down despite excellent wound care, worsening labs (such as tumor markers or organ function tests), or increasing visits to the doctor or hospital.

The above guidelines are a partial list of the most common symptoms for the most common illnesses that bring patients to hospice. Hopefully the information is not too technical (a difficult task, especially with HIV). With this information we hope that patients who wish to explore the hospice option will have the basis for an informed discussion with their physician regarding possible hospice referral. This information is critical for you to have because unless your physician is board certified in hospice and palliative medicine, it is unlikely that he is familiar with the qualifying details for hospice referral in these disease categories. For you, the patient or caregiver, in what may seem the darkest and most stressful time of your life, this information should give you hope that there are options, there is help, and there is wonderful and abundant support awaiting you with hospice.

Silent Night

Mid-December, a couple of years ago, my wife and I brought up dozens of boxes of Christmas decorations from the basement. Exhausted, we plopped down on the couch to take a break. Scanning over all the memories we had collected in our thirty-five Christmases together, we recalled some of our favorite ones. We talked of our first Christmas together and then of the ones of when the kids were small. The joyful nostalgia was flavored with a bit of sadness realizing this was the first Christmas with all of our parents gone.

This had been my mom's favorite time of the year. Not only was it Christmas time, which she had always relished as a teacher and principal, but her birthday was three days after Christmas as well. As a devout Christian, she rejoiced in the "reason for the season" and loved to play the piano and sing carols at home and at church. One of her favorite possessions was a music-box ornament she had received as a gift from my grandparents when she was a child that played "Silent Night" when the string was pulled. We still had the ornament, but unfortunately since Mom died, the string had gotten stuck and the song would no longer play.

As we sat there talking about her and her ornament, I began to miss her terribly. Then suddenly, from deep within one of the boxes, the sweet, clear strains of the familiar song began to rise. I rushed to the boxes, and after finding the right one, I dug down and pulled out the ancient red globe that had entranced my mother as a child. The tempo slowed as the string disappeared one last time. Thanks, Mom. Merry Christmas. I miss you too.

3

CHARTING YOUR COURSE
WITH ADVANCE DIRECTIVES

Long before the subject of hospice, or even chronic illness, is a concern, all people over the age of eighteen years,
should have a record of their wishes regarding health care
decisions. In the event of people's inability to express their
own wishes, the document needs to state whom they have
chosen to make health care decisions on their behalf and
their health care preferences.

The best way to ensure that each patient's wishes will
be honored is to create a document known as the patient's
"Advance Health Care Directive" (AHCD) or living will.
The most important reason for completing an AHCD is to
name a person as your health care decision maker should
you be unable to make the decisions on your own. The second reason *is* to clearly document your wishes beforehand:
you can make your wishes known regarding such issues
as circumstances where you would want resuscitation,

tube feeding, blood transfusions, certain medical treatments or procedures, organ donation, or donation of your body for scientific research or medical education, and so on. Although some of the specific laws and regulations vary from state to state, advance directives are recognized nationwide.

In preparation for the completion of this document, you should discuss the various options with your physician and your family. It is important to emphasize that this document is *patient centered*; it conveys the wishes of the individual creating it. It does not give the designated surrogate decision maker the permission or right to impose one's own wishes or values on the course of treatment if the patient becomes incapacitated.

When an eligible patient enrolls in hospice, the team needs to design a plan of care to manage the specific needs of the patient. We need to know what the goals of the patient are so that we may assist in making the patient's remaining time the best it can be. Decisions need to be made and documented so the plan of care can be created. Some patients are too impaired or too close to death to be able to participate in decision making. However, the ones who are able to communicate need to be asked about the issues that are the most important to them in making their remaining lives meaningful and the things that give them the greatest sense of choice and control in managing their end-of-life experience.

It is important to understand that ethnic and cultural background may influence the plan of care. Treatment choices as well as decision-maker roles should not be assumed by the hospice team but rather should be established after detailed discussion with the patient and family. Some people do not want to know about the complicated or distressing details of their health and delegate the decision making to a family member or surrogate. It is important that a patient chooses a surrogate decision maker who is able to follow their wishes, knows their preferences, can make difficult decisions, is available, and will speak for the patient even against their own interests and beliefs.

A challenge that we may have in patient decision making is that the primary physician withholds distressing information from the patient or family regarding the gravity of their condition or their expected survival time. This may arise from a feeling of compassion, not wanting to take away the patient's hope, or perhaps even due to personal issues the physician has with the subject of death.

Communication also breaks down when family physicians feel that it is the responsibility of one of the patient's specialists to speak to the issue of prognosis, as new drugs, procedures, and research results are coming out at a very fast pace. But when the specialists feel their only job is to report their findings and recommendations to the primary physician, the difficult talk with the patient and family may not happen until very late in the disease. It is impossible to make *informed* decisions about care at the end of life if the patient and family are not fully aware of the patient's condition, expected course of action, treatment options, and the respective burdens and benefits of each course of action.

The road map for the patient's end-of-life care is based on the patient's, or their decision maker's, fully informed understanding of the patient's conditions, prognosis, and options as well as the patient's goals, values, and quality of life. From these two guideposts, we create the hospice plan of care. The care plan takes the form of the medical orders that document specific choices of treatment at the end of life. To summarize these wishes and make them easily accessible and transportable, they are often in the form of a document called the POLST or MOLST form. This acronym stands for "physician (or medical) orders for life sustaining treatment."

This form is entirely voluntary, not mandatory for hospice enrollment, and may vary somewhat from state to state. It may be called by a variety of other names. This record of the patient's wishes is signed by the patient (or their surrogate decision-making designee) as well as their health care provider. Although a copy of this document may go in the chart, the original is intended to stay in the possession of the patient, so first responders, and any facility to which the patient is transported, have the original signed wishes of the patient.

The form should be filled out by the patient with the aid of trained medical staff, as it requires a detailed discussion with the patient and/or family about what these choices mean and why these questions are being asked. It needs to be clear to anyone signing for the patient that the form is expressing the wishes of the patient, not the wishes of another person who is signing the form. The POLST form in California can only be signed by the patient (if they have the mental capacity to do so) or the designated surrogate decision maker who appears on the AHCD. Check online for the requirements of your particular state or jurisdiction.

Frequently, family members will feel they are "betraying" a parent if they "stop fighting for recovery" or limit care in any way. What needs to be made clear is that they are signing an attestation of what the patient expressed to them, as to what their wishes are, or what their wishes would be, if they could still make their own decision. It is not betrayal to make sure a patient's wishes are carried out; it is a betrayal to put them through additional suffering by not putting their wishes first. We often come across family members and caregivers who have been compassionately advocating for their loved one through a long and frustrating battle with their illness. It may be difficult for them to pivot from the position "We can't just give up!" or "We can't just let him die!" This is where reassurance needs to be given that further treatment would likely just mean further suffering.

In hospice, we understand that we should not fear death but, rather, embrace its inevitability. In the great cycle of life, physical death, which ends all physical suffering, is as essential to this cycle as is birth. Allowing the body to naturally do its orderly and soothing process of shutting down is a logical and compassionate option at the end of life. Hospice chaplains are nonsectarian and trained to address any existential concerns regarding death, for all patients, religious or not. If the patient or family wishes, the chaplain can help to coordinate visits by a minister, priest, or imam of the patient's choosing.

Often, the most difficult decision for families is whether to attempt CPR/resuscitation or not, when the heart stops. If the terminal illness, or another severe chronic illness afflicting the patient, is the cause of cardiac arrest, it is essential to provide education to the family that the patient has a disease that will only get worse. CPR will not lessen the disease or make it go away. With terminal disease–related death, CPR is not only medically ineffective but it may also cause the patient further suffering. Organs are often damaged or ruptured, and fragile ribs can be crushed. And, in the extremely unlikely event of temporarily restoring a heartbeat, there is only the guarantee that the heart will soon stop again. Allowing natural death to occur may bring final, permanent relief and peace and comfort to their loved one.

Regarding the intensity of treatment, full treatment means all the aggressive care that the hospital has to offer will be attempted. This is rarely the choice of hospice patients, as this choice prioritizes prolonging life by artificial means, regardless of the suffering that this may cause. Patients and families may choose this if physical life prolongation is their highest priority, regardless of the suffering it causes. However, this goal is not consistent with hospice philosophy. If further discussions with the patient and/or family indicate that they want life prolongation at any cost, they may not be psychologically ready for hospice, and a palliative care program may be more appropriate for the time being.

The second choice, "selective treatment," is for hospice patients early in the course of their terminal illness who are still experiencing an adequate quality of life that allows them to enjoy their families and friends as well as finish up financial or legal matters before they become incapacitated. Various medical treatments including IV fluids, external respiratory support (such as BiPAP), blood products, and/or antibiotics can be used to restore the patient's temporary base-line function before the inevitable final decline.

When maintaining a state of adequately comfortable function is no longer possible, the third choice is "comfort-focused treatment." With this choice, comfort is prioritized over function, even if the moment of death comes sooner. Most people would not choose a few more hours or days of life if pain is the only thing keeping them going. This is a frequent choice for almost all hospice patients who are late in the course of their disease. Anything more than the alleviation of suffering would simply increase this suffering and just prolong the dying process.

Sometimes situations arise that require a judgment call. Hip fractures due to falls are not uncommon. If the patient is relatively active and has months to live, surgery to stabilize the painful fracture is reasonable. If the patient is near death, the pain can be managed with medications, and without surgery. The focus should be on what will allow the patient to have the most comfortable and functional time.

Artificially administered nutrition is another treatment decision to be considered. Again, most hospice patients select the choice of "No artificial means of nutrition," but many may want to attempt life prolongation with fluid and nutritional support for cultural, religious, or personal reasons. In these cases, any worsening or prolongation of end-of-life symptoms may be managed in other ways. For some, this is a difficult choice, as we frequently hear families say that they do not want their family member to die of hunger or thirst. What these families may not know is that the loss of the desire for food and water is part of a natural progression leading to death. If hunger and thirst are gone, it is impossible to die of something that you do not have.

The body, in its wisdom, dials down the sensations of hunger and thirst at the end of life for very good reasons. When the body is about to transition through death, it is the *lack* of fluid and nutrition that brings about metabolic changes that not only relieve suffering but also, according to many who believe so, bring about euphoria and spiritual clarity that prepare the patient for what is beyond— more on this in a later chapter. But, at the very end of life, forcing the artificial intake of nutrition and fluid will almost always increase suffering and prolong the active-dying process. We recognize that in some cultures it may be important for the patient to have something in their stomach for the journey after death.

The AHCD is essential in establishing *a surrogate decision maker*, a patient-centered plan of care, and assuring that the patient will have their wishes honored. An AHCD can only be completed by a patient who has mental decision-making capacity. This is why every capable person over the age of 18 should complete one. A guideline for end-of-life orders (such as a POLST) can be completed by the decision maker designated in the AHCD of an incapacitated patient. If a patient has a legal conservator, that person may complete a form for end-of-life orders. The plan of care is not intended to represent the wishes of the surrogate decision maker. Only the patient's wishes (or presumed wishes) are part of a plan of treatment for the patient.

The simple loving act of making sure a loved-one's final wishes are honored, whether you agree with them or not, should give one a sense of pride, not guilt. The patient's wishes are the moral issue of the patient alone; there is no moral burden on the messenger. It should also be remembered that when someone loves you and trusts you enough to make some of the most profound decisions of their life on their behalf, there may be no higher honor that one can bestow.

Tapping

Trudy told me that of all the personal relationships in her life, the strongest connection she ever had was with her mother. Trudy, one of our hospice nurses, was very concerned about her mother, who lived in another state, and who was terminally ill. One night, at exactly 7:03 p.m., she heard three distinct taps on her upstairs bedroom window. Intuitively, she knew immediately that it was her mother telling her that she was finally free of her pain. She suddenly felt a great sense of peace that Mom had let her know that she had passed and that she was OK and no longer suffering. At 7:08 p.m., the phone rang. It was her father calling to notify her of her mother's passing, just five minutes earlier. "I know, Dad," Trudy said as she smiled through the tears, "I know."

"I figured you would," he replied with a smile.

4

MANAGING PAIN

Probably the greatest fear for patients facing death is the amount of suffering they will be going through. Adequate pain management is always at the top of the list for symptom management for hospice physicians. Fortunately, our bag of tricks is very deep. One of the factors that makes pain management such a challenge is the fact that pain is a subjective experience. It is what the patient feels. This makes it even more challenging managing pain in a patient who is not verbal or is confused. The physician often needs to rely heavily on the reports of the family when determining what pain medication to use and when to change the dose. This chapter will attempt to help the family identify the presence of pain along with its severity and give some tips on what is, and is not, helpful in managing pain in the home.

There are different types of pain. How the patient experiences the pain may depend on a number of factors.

Pain is usually caused by healthy nerves detecting damage or a threat of damage to the body. This is known as "nociceptive pain." Pain can also be caused by sick or damaged nerves sending false pain signals to the brain. This is called "neuropathic pain" (common in diabetes and many other diseases). The perception of pain can be amplified by anxiety, depression, family discord, spiritual and existential issues, or sensory deprivation. Besides the use of medications, pain can be diminished by distraction, improving mood, providing hope for pain relief, guided imagery, hypnosis, music therapy, or even providing medications or treatments that the patient *believes* will relieve pain but actually have no pharmacologic effect (the placebo effect). The same amount of stimulation to a pain nerve can go unnoticed or cause severe distress. This is why we try to determine the difference between the stimulation of certain nerves (pain) and the reaction to this stimulation (suffering). This is difficult as pain is a "whole person experience" which not only affects the patient's body but all aspects of a person's life and relationships as well.

It can be challenging to know if someone is in pain when they cannot communicate verbally. However, we do have a few nonverbal indicators of pain that can be quite useful. For example, (remember this one!) if a patient with dementia becomes *combative,* often with restlessness, increased pulse, blood pressure, or respirations, increased vocalizations and grimacing, he or she is likely to be in pain. Do not first go for antipsychotics such as haloperidol (Haldol) or quetiapine (Seroquel). If possible, assess the patient for the source of the pain (one of our patients had a thumbtack through the bottom of his slipper). Remove, correct, or resolve the cause of the discomfort if possible and see if this solves the problem. If the cause of the behavior is pain, but it cannot be identified, or cannot be corrected, first try medicating the patient for pain. If symptoms resolve, pain was likely the reason for the behavior. (More on agitation and delirium in a later chapter.)

Pain management is less challenging when the patient is coherent and verbal. The location and cause of the source of pain is much easier to identify. RICE (rest, ice, compression, elevation) is the usual recommendation for trauma-induced pain. Chronic painful areas often respond to intermittent ice or heat, or topical liniments mimic those sensations containing capsaicin or menthol (Bengay, Icy Hot, etc.). If over-the-counter oral medication is used, acetaminophen (Tylenol) is preferred unless the patient has severe liver disease. Lower doses are now recommended (no more than 3,000 mg/day; 2,400 mg/day in the elderly, and even less with liver disease).

Nonsteroidal anti-inflammatory drugs (NSAIDs) like ibuprophen (Advil) or naproxen (Aleve) can cause stomach upset and side effects that are more severe in the elderly. NSAIDs can cause GI bleeding, severe kidney failure, confusion, constipation, dry mouth, and inability to empty the bladder, to name a few things. They also should never be taken with steroids (Prednisone, Decadron, etc.) as they compete for the same pathways and greatly increase the risk of internal bleeding. Topical NSAIDs are easier on the stomach but work by being absorbed into the general circulation. They need not be applied to the painful area. Lidocaine patches (Lidoderm, Salonpas, etc.) only numb skin nerves such as for the pain after an infection with shingles. They are expensive and unlikely to be useful for arthritic pain, low back pain, or other sources of pain that are separated from the skin by several layers of tissue. Any perceived benefit is placebo. Duct tape is cheaper and equally effective.

Notify your doctor if the patient is depressed (the best test for this is asking "Are you depressed?"—seriously). Also, tearfulness, withdrawal from social interaction or hobbies and recreation, hopelessness, inability to experience pleasure, early morning wakening, and decreased appetite may also be signs of depression. Not only can depression worsen the experience of pain, it is an independent risk factor for mortality, that is, a depressed person is likely to die sooner than a nondepressed person with the same condition. Medications to treat depression commonly reduce suffering for any type of pain but especially for neuropathic pain. Medications for anxiety can be useful as well either by themselves or in combination with antidepressants and/or pain medications.

When the pain is intermittent or not very severe, prescription pain medications can be given as needed. As the disease progresses and the pain worsens and becomes constantly present, it is advisable to keep the pain away with scheduled pain medication. In patients who cannot communicate and become more agitated, even a trial of scheduled Tylenol may give a clue whether or not the agitation is caused by pain. Scheduling short-acting pain medications becomes problematic as they may only last four to six hours and may need someone to give them around the clock. Extended release pain medications usually last at least twelve hours. The goal is to have the patient's pain controlled most of the time but still use short-acting medication two to three times a day for breakthrough pain.

Opioid-based pain medication (drugs created based on the structure of the opium molecule) are the mainstay of hospice pain control. These include such medications as morphine (tablets or the liquid concentrate Roxanol), hydromorphone (Dilaudid), hydrocodone (Vicodin, Norco, and others), codeine, oxycodone, methadone, and others. We try to avoid the use of fentanyl because of its widely variable and changeable absorption, difficulty in calculating alternative equivalent dosages, potentially fatal diversion and abuse potential, as well as cost. These medications are relatively inexpensive in their short acting form, have few side effects, and rarely cause true allergic reactions.

Side effects may include itching, drowsiness, nausea and vomiting, confusion, hallucinations, and constipation. Morphine, which is mostly cleared from the body by the kidneys, should be used cautiously in patients with impaired kidneys, and avoided in patients with severe kidney failure. In patients requiring very high doses of morphine, especially ones with kidney disease, toxic break-down products of morphine can build up, which can cause muscle jerking, and can actually increase the patient's pain.

Combination medications, where the opiate is combined with acetaminophen (Tylenol) or ibuprophen, such as Tylenol with codeine, Norco, Vicodin, Percocet, Roxicet, Vicoprophen, and such, may have some limited use early in the hospice course but become toxic when higher doses are needed. Uncompounded pain medication allows much safer dosage increases and reduces confusion if the patient starts having side effects.

One of the great things about opiates is that the dose can be increased until pain control is achieved. There is no upper limit or maximum dose. For a long-acting pain medication, we mostly use methadone (methadone should not be used by physicians who are not trained in its use and peculiarities). Methadone doses can last as little as six hours in the young and healthy and as long as eighty hours in the elderly. Because of its prolonged action, very low doses are given, which "stack" on each other over three to seven days before equilibrium is achieved. Dosage increases should be done no more often than every four to seven days. The prescribing physician should be aware of potential risks, (QT interval prolongation) for one, drug interactions (SSRIs, etc.), and the potential for delayed signs of overdose.

But the risks of methadone are certainly worth the benefits. Tiny volumes per dose of the 10mg/ml solution allow oral absorption even when the patient can no longer swallow. Methadone stands alone among the opiates in its effectiveness with treating neuropathic pain of damaged nerves, not just nociceptive pain of intact nerves registering danger or tissue injury. The long half-life (how long the body takes to remove half the drug from the circulation) provides consistent pain control and reduces the rollercoaster over-sedation-then-breakthrough of shorter acting drugs.

We have another superstar of pain control that we use for cancer pain. That drug is a steroid called dexamethasone (Decadron). Because the body reacts to cancer as something foreign, cancers can cause system-wide inflammatory reactions, excruciating increases of pressure inside bones, increased pressure on the brain (when cancer is present inside the skull), and blockages of intestines and other hollow organs in the body. Dexamethasone reduces this inflammation and swelling, providing at times tremendous reduction in suffering. As a bonus, dexamethasone can improve mood (which also reduces suffering), improves appetite, reduces fluid accumulation in the abdomen and/or chest cavities, and can open up not only some early intestinal obstructions but airways as well. With its forty-eight-hour half-life, it only needs to be taken once daily, with food, in the morning (so it doesn't interfere with sleep). The dose can be split and given with breakfast and lunch if the whole dose upsets the stomach. Acid blockers should be given as well, and again, *no NSAIDs while on steroids*!

Another class of adjunctive medications we use for pain control is the neurostimulant category. Drugs like methylphenidate (Ritalin) and amphetamines (Dexedrine, Adderall, etc.) can assist in several ways. First, they appear to directly enhance the effectiveness of other pain medications. They improve mood by acting as an antidepressant, which reduces suffering, and improves alertness and focus, as well as reducing the fatigue that pain medications can cause. The down side is that they can occasionally cause loss of appetite, stomach pain, insomnia, anxiety or irritability, rapid heart rate, or elevation in blood pressure. It is best to take these medications just in the morning or morning and early afternoon.

The problems with pain medications include overuse in patients with a history of substance abuse, and theft or sale of drugs by family members, caregivers or visitors. For this reason, caregivers should treat the controlled drugs the same way they would treat cash. Keep controlled drugs secured and out of sight. Concerns about accidental overdose are largely unfounded when medications are given as prescribed by experienced practitioners. The amount of opiate medication that will completely relieve symptoms is only a fraction of the amount it would take to kill the patient.

The patient will pass away no matter what you do. The only way the last dose of pain medication will affect the moment of the patient's death is if their pain is the only thing keeping them breathing. Prolonging the agony of dying is far worse than allowing the body to comfortably shut down with adequate pain control. The appropriate use of pain medication in terminal illness does not create addiction behaviors. In forty years of medicine, I have never had a hospice patient have a decline in morality, start associating with the "wrong crowd", or "knock over" a liquor store. People who come to hospice with addictive personalities can occasionally be a problem, but adequate supervision, support, and symptom control make big problems rare.

Terminal illnesses, especially cancer, can create profound pain problems. Fortunately, we have profound solutions to these problems. For example, if a spinal tumor is crushing the spinal cord causing excruciating pain and new onset paralysis, palliative radiation can be amazingly effective in relieving suffering and restoring function in patients not yet in the active-dying stage. What's more, depending on where exactly the tumor is, seven difficult and painful visits may not be necessary for the course of radiation. Hypo-fractionated single dose radiation gives all the radiation at once and may result in the same benefit achieved by daily radiation for a week.

Oral pain medication takes only one hour to reach maximum blood levels. Subcutaneous injection under the skin takes only a half hour to reach maximum blood levels, and intravenous injections reach maximum levels in only ten to fifteen minutes. Intramuscular injections are no longer used because of increased pain of administration and variability of absorption. Two-thirds of the oral dose does not make it to the general circulation. So, for the same effect, the oral dose must be three times higher than the injected dose. For patients who no longer are taking anything orally, a relatively new device, the Macy catheter, can be placed rectally for medication administration. The absorption of medication is quite rapid and blood levels may peak in as little as twenty minutes. If the medication from a pump is fed by a catheter into the spinal canal (epidural), it takes only a tenth of the injected dose for the same effect. If the medication is introduced directly into the spinal fluid (intra-thecal) via a catheter from a medication reservoir in a pump implanted inside the abdominal cavity, it requires only one-tenth of the epidural dose. This means that the same dose that relieves the pain by being given directly inside the coverings of the spinal cord is three hundred times more effective than if it were given by mouth.

Besides implanted pain pumps and palliative radiation, anesthesiologists can block or destroy the pain nerves in the abdominal cavity coming from severely painful tumor areas. In addition, there are new pain medication coming out all the time as well as new uses for old medications such as ketamine (until recently mainly a veterinary anesthetic). Acupuncture, mindfulness/meditation, and many other things are being studied for use for end of life suffering.

But what do we do when the burdens and side effects of comfort care seem too much to bear and the end of life is on a distant horizon? Although physician-assisted suicide is legal in some states, the vast majority of physicians refuse to participate in the program. Most feel that the only moral justification for taking (or participating in taking) an innocent human life is when doing so would save many others, and there are no other options. For most people who chose the physician-assisted suicide option, it is not for what they are going through but fear of what they might go through. In addition, there are those who "do not want to be a burden" or "sacrifice their dignity" to their children who were "a burden" to them for years, changing their diapers and feeding them. There are also the highest suicide risk group of "old white guys" who either think their illness will bankrupt the family that they spent a lifetime trying to make financially secure or have "nothing to live for" after becoming widowers.

By understanding the myriad of options of hospice that allow the body to naturally shut down, and getting the counseling, support, and medications for depression if needed, patients can allow the hospice team to work with them in their concerns. There is a reason that for twenty-five hundred years we physicians have abided by the words of the Hippocratic Oath, "I will not give poison if asked to do so, nor will I suggest such a course." Let's look at the less sardonic options.

Patients on hospice have the right to discontinue medication that are extending their lives. Insulin and cardiac and respiratory medications as well as antibiotics can be discontinued and whatever symptoms arise can be treated with comfort medications. In addition, medical devices such as CPAP, BiPAP, nebulizers, pacemaker, and defibrillator can be discontinued. The patient can voluntarily stop eating and drinking. This also could be made quite tolerable with hospice comfort medications. Finally, if all else fails, and symptom management can be achieved no other way, we utilize palliative sedation. With this option we use sedative medications such as lorazepam, morphine and/ or phenobarbital adjusted to a rate or frequency where the patient is still alive and breathing but unable to experience any of their symptoms. Similar medications are used as the ones with physician-assisted suicide, but at nonlethal dosages.

Sir, Yes, Sir!

Mac was well into his eighties when he came under our care. Lisa was his hospice nurse case manager. He had widespread prostate cancer, yet he was still able to mostly care for himself and still having mostly good days. Despite his current status, his cancer doctor felt his time on hospice would be short due to how aggressive his disease was.

Mac had spent thirty years in the US Army. His ramrod posture, spit-and-polish appearance, and solemn demeanor were as just as much a part of him as were his heart, brain, and kidneys. His home was a museum of military memorabilia—a tribute to a life of service to his country and his travels around the world. Despite the display of his extensive achievements, he rarely spoke of his service experiences and never of his times in combat.

The first thing he wanted to know about Lisa was if she had ever been in the military. She was proud to tell him of her seven years of active duty and seven more in the reserves. He simply nodded and said, Good, and never brought the issue up again. Still, Lisa felt a bond had been forged between them, far deeper than their few words to each other seemed to show.

Soon however, the burden of his advancing disease and the powerful medications needed to manage his terminal symptoms released in him the demons of his past from the living nightmare of his combat experiences. The desperate warrior's fierce resistance to the foes in his body and mind resulted in behaviors that could no longer be managed in the home.

Now heavily sedated in the hospital, Lisa's morning visit found him finally peaceful in a deep coma. As she sat at his bedside, holding his hand, she silently thanked him for letting her be a part of his care. She strongly felt from him an echo of gratitude for the care he received. As he was very near death, she could not help but whisper, So, soldier, when are you shipping out?

A startling response came to her as clear as if he were speaking out loud, Around four. As she regained her composure, she smiled, made sure he was comfortable, and with a final farewell salute she left the room. As she would not have time to get back to the hospital that afternoon, she knew she would not see him again.

At the end of the day she checked her phone for any messages regarding him passing. No word on Mac. Although it seemed so real, her silent communication with her valiant comrade must have been only in her overactive imagination.

The next morning a voice mail on her phone reported that Mac had just died around 4:00 a.m. that morning. Somewhat surprised that he didn't pass at 4:00 p.m. yesterday, a stern but familiar voice rang in her head, "If I had meant sixteen hundred, I would have said, 'Sixteen hundred'!" Sir, yes, sir!

5

MANAGING CONSTIPATION AND DIARRHEA

Opiate pain medication is the first line of defense against the number one problem in hospice symptom management—pain. This brings us to the number one side effect of this number one treatment for the number one problem, which is constipation. (Constipation can be a problem for hospice patients who are not on pain medications as well.) Prevention and treatment of constipation must be individualized. Normal bowel patterns vary from one person to another. Some people have multiple bowel movements a day, others as infrequently as once a week. As age advances, constipation can become more of an issue even without opiates. In addition to normal aging, medications play more of a part in bowel irregularity. With advancing age comes advancing symptoms as organ systems decline and fail, and aches and pains become a constant companion of the elderly.

Constipation can be not only a major problem in itself but the cause of many other problems as well. The longer constipation goes unaddressed, the more trouble it can cause. First of all, it can kill an already fragile appetite or even cause vomiting. Constipation is a major factor when it comes to feeding. If there is nowhere for the food to go, the body loses its desire for it. If the stool (poop) sits in the rectum for long, it becomes so hard and dry that it forms a blockage that the patient cannot pass on their own, called an impaction. This hard blockage can press forward and pinch the urethra (the tube that drains urine from the bladder) against the inside edge of the pubic bone causing the bladder to overstretch and cause severe distress, or simply keep the bladder from emptying, resulting in infections, kidney failure, confusion, agitation, lethargy, and poor intake, including dehydration. The hard blockage can also cause "overflow diarrhea," which may not be recognized as severe constipation resulting in the wrong treatment.

We cared for a man with advanced rectal cancer that was not diagnosed until late in the disease process. When we first saw him at the facility, he had been suffering from diarrhea for weeks. The facility protocol was to administer Imodium for his diarrhea. This made no difference to his watery loose stools. A careful assessment by the hospice staff revealed a large rectal mass narrowing the bowel and a hard-impacted stool above the mass. He had "overflow diarrhea." We started him on Dexamethasone, a bowel stimulant, and gave him three pea-size Vaseline balls to lubricate the hard stool. He eventually passed the stool. We then ensured very soft frequent stools were passed daily.

Medications that never were a problem when the patient was younger can become much more of a problem as the patient ages. Medications take longer to clear from the system in the elderly and side effects become more common. Many medications have a set of side effects that can be very problematic in the elderly. These are drugs that have *anticholinergic (AC)* side effects, that is, they interfere with the normal functioning of the bladder, the bowels, the salivary glands, and tear formation. They also can cause drowsiness, falls, confusion, agitation, psychosis, and heart rhythm and blood pressure problems. These medications include the older antihistamines (Benadryl, etc.), over-the-counter sleep aids (anything "PM"), older antidepressants (Elavil/amitriptyline, etc.), some muscle relaxers, and anti-inflammatory pain relievers (NSAIDs) like Advil (ibuprofen) or Aleve (naproxen), as well as many others. The problems that AC medications cause are worse when more than one is used at the same time (such as Aleve PM, a combination of naproxen and the active ingredient in Benadryl).

Normal bowel function is supported by adequate fiber intake, adequate fluid intake, and exercise. The stomach and intestines rhythmically squeeze food and fluid toward the rectum. With aging, disease, and medication, food and fluid intake diminish, and activity declines. While the AC medications slow down the bowels, opiate pain medications can shut bowel activity down much more. This is why it is a hospice policy to always start a bowel medication that stimulates the squeezing action of the bowels. Stool softeners like docusate (Colace) can make stools softer but do nothing to restore the squeezing activity that moves things through the intestines. Metamucil can actually cause constipation if the patient does not take in enough water. Senna and Bisacodyl (Dulcolax) are the mainstays of bowel care in patients on opiate pain medication. Bisacodyl also comes in a rectal suppository. Senna is a natural vegetable-based bowel stimulant. Bisacodyl also stimulates the squeezing action of the bowels but is a drug.

When there is a hard impaction of stool in the rectum that the patient cannot pass, it may first need to be partially removed by *gently* digging it out with your gloved finger. Oil enemas lubricate the dry stool and can help the patient pass the rest of it. Saline or water enemas can help the process by softening the stool. When the bowel is overstretched, it loses its strength to squeeze things through. Often, after stool is removed from the rectum by hand or enema, a bisacodyl suppository may help greatly in restoring the bowel's normal size and function.

Due to the potential risk of severe kidney, heart, and metabolic problems, we no longer recommend phosphosoda enemas (Fleets, etc.). Fleets does make oil and saline enemas as well that are safe. We do not recommend oral mineral oil as it may get into the lungs when swallowing becomes more of a problem. Milk of magnesia and magnesium citrate can be a problem in patients with kidney failure (as oral intake diminishes, all patients have reduced kidney function). If the patient can take the fluid volume required, polyethylene glycol (MiraLAX, etc.) can be very useful in resolving constipation by holding water in the intestinal tract (osmotic laxative).

As death approaches, the intestinal tract is one of the first systems to shut down. If little or no food or fluids is entering the GI tract, you cannot expect anything to come out. (We often use the analogy that if no cars are going into the tunnel, no cars will come out of the tunnel.) Just make sure you are not dealing with an impaction. Forcing bowel movements with overly aggressive use of bowel medications, when the patient is not eating and near death, not only can cause pain and distress for the patient, the extra movement of the patient required for changing and cleaning can cause quite a bit of suffering. In addition, prolonged contact of stool with the skin causes the skin to become inflamed and quickly break down.

Diarrhea is usually less of a problem. But before using over-the-counter remedies, contact your physician to make him aware of the situation. It is best to first know the cause of the diarrhea and treat the cause of it. Some diarrhea related to antibiotic use (Clostridium Difficile or "C. Diff") can result in severe illness and death if the infected stool is not expelled from the body. Some antibiotics are worse than others for risk of C. Diff. Steroids (Prednisone, Decadron, etc.) and acid blockers (Prilosec, Nexium, etc.), greatly increase the risk of C. Diff when given with certain antibiotics.

If C. Diff has been ruled out, the patient is not severely constipated with overflow diarrhea, and the diarrhea is new in onset, clear liquids and bland starches are the least likely to aggravate the diarrhea. Citrus and dairy are particularly bad when the intestine is inflamed. If the diarrhea is chronic or longstanding, over-the-counter remedies such as Imodium or Lomotil may decrease the frequency of soiling. Bulk-forming fiber agents such as Metamucil may be helpful in absorbing excess intestinal fluid and slowing overactive bowels. If the issue becomes a major problem, your physician may shut off bowel fluid production all together with octreotide injections. Sometimes an impaction may be blocking the rectum and liquid stool leaking around it. If this is the case, medication for diarrhea will just compound the problem. Always check for impaction prior to starting diarrhea medication, especially in a hospice patient who is at much higher risk for constipation than for diarrhea.

Koi

After Doc Wilson finally hung up his stethoscope, he immersed himself in his passion—Koi fish ponds. He spent his retirement constructing three elegant koi ponds in his backyard and two in his front yard. He loved the beautiful multicolored creatures that gave him such a feeling of peace and harmony in our often violent and chaotic world. As he neared the end of his life on hospice, his hospital bed was moved to where the dining room table had been because that was the only room that had large picture window views of all the ponds in both the front yard the and backyard. The views of his beloved fish brought him as much comfort and peace as any of our medications.

The weekly case review meeting finally came when Doc Wilson's name appeared on the list of deaths in the past week. One of the case manager nurses, Alita, was at his bedside when he passed. She presented his case in the usual fashion, but then added, "You know what was really strange? At the moment that he took his last breath, all the fish in all the ponds began leaping out of the water. I didn't know they did that."

Maybe they don't do that for everyone, only the ones they love.

6

MANAGING SHORTNESS OF BREATH

Shortness of breath is one of the worst symptoms that someone can experience. Unfortunately, it is one of the most common symptoms we have to deal with in hospice. Patients with chronic lung disease or heart disease experience this symptom from quite early in their illness. Patients with neurodegenerative disorders, such as muscular dystrophy, ALS (Lou Gehrig's Disease), or multiple sclerosis, experience worsening of difficulty breathing every day. Cancers can either replace normal lung tissue or fill the chest cavity with cancerous fluid, compressing the lungs. Cancers cause the blood to become more likely to cause clots in the veins, which often break off and find their way to the lungs, blocking oxygen-starved blood from getting access to the air. Infections, kidney failure, and diabetes can cause the buildup of acid in the blood, triggering rapid breathing. Massive amounts of fluid can fill the abdominal cavity in liver failure and compress the diaphragm, causing respiratory distress. Any chronic illness can cause poor nutrition or leave the body unable to utilize the nutrition that it gets, resulting in low albumen levels (the protein that draws fluid out of the tissues and into the blood vessels), allowing fluid to collect in the lungs (pulmonary edema). This last situation is most common in cases where misguided efforts to artificially force fluid and nutrition into a body whose hunger and thirst have long gone. Also, patients may become anemic (low number of red blood cells) and feel short of breath because not enough oxygen can be delivered to the body.

Fortunately, we have many tools to deal with this problem. The first step we take is for optimum medical management, with the goal not to prolong life but rather reduce symptoms. The use of water pills for fluid overload are commonly used. If fluid is accumulating in the chest cavity or abdominal cavity, the patient can be sent at hospice expense to the interventional radiologist to have this fluid drained off. If the accumulation of fluid is frequent, drainage tubes can be placed so the patient can have the fluid drained at home. Cancer patients who initially ask how long they can have artificial feeding and fluid by IVs soon request to stop as their lungs become more congested and the natural soothing end-of-life chemicals that the body produces have been flushed out of the system by the forced fluid overload. Blood clots in the lungs can be dissolved by blood thinners. Massively elevated blood sugars causing acid buildup can be brought down to levels that do not cause symptoms.

As far as dealing directly with the breathing problem, there are external assistive devices, such as BiPAP and CPAP, that can aid in the mechanical aspect of breathing when the muscles are too weak to do the necessary work of breathing, thus extending temporarily the time of acceptable comfort and function. If it is a true deficiency of oxygen that is causing the discomfort, oxygen supplementation can be administered. However, most of the time, the same relief from shortness of breath can be achieved with simply having a fan blowing on the face or a cool wash cloth applied to the face. When death is near and the patient is unresponsive or actively dying, oxygen supplementation can only make the patient more aware of their suffering and prolong the dying process. At this point, relief is best achieved by medications.

There comes a time when the artificial intervention of external breathing support begins to cause more suffering and distress than it relieves. As an example, we had a wonderful patient, we will call him Chris, a young man in his thirties, who had ALS (Lou Gehrig's Disease). He was brilliant and funny and had to retire from his exciting career in the entertainment industry due to his disease. He had a very supportive and loving family who took meticulous care of him. However, his disease had progressed to the point where he increasingly could no longer notify them of any of his needs or if he was in any distress.

About a year prior, he chose to artificially extend his life by using an external breathing-assistive device. This allowed him to enjoy his relationships with his family and friends for many months more than he could without it. But now, he could no longer enjoy life; it had become a burden. Due to his progressive weakness, he was soon to be cut off from any communication with his family. Before his ability to choose for himself was gone and awful burden of this decision fell on his family, he decided to have his brother discontinue the breathing-assist device on his thirty-eighth birthday, "so my mom would grieve my loss only one day a year."

The challenge was finding a way to remain comfortable while he died of respiratory failure off the machine. He had his family contact us. Jim and I went out to his house and spoke with him and the family about their goals. Chris had chosen this intervention to extend his life, and he made the informed decision to discontinue it. We discussed the options and decided on palliative sedation. We would administer IV sedation just to the point where he would be unable to experience any suffering; then in compliance with Chris's wishes, his brother would turn off the breathing machine. It would be his disease, not the medication or his brother's actions, that would take his life, months after he should have died.

We arrived the day of his birthday. His family and friends were there. He had incense burning and his favorite music playing. We started the IV and soon he was sleeping and unresponsive to any pain. When the family was ready, his brother turned off and removed the machine. Within the hour Chris peacefully crossed over, with his angelic face still reflecting his love for his family. It was an honor to know him.

Opiate pain medications are the go-to drugs in relief of shortness of breath. The doses need only be about half of what would be given for pain. The relief usually lasts around twice as long as well. Morphine and hydromorphone (Dilaudid) are the ones most commonly used. Methadone does not seem to be particularly effective in treating shortness of breath. As the disease progresses and difficulty breathing increases, higher doses of medication can be given as needed, with no upper limit except that of symptom relief. Again, it takes a dose many times higher to stop someone's breathing than it does to completely relieve symptoms. The only exception to this is if the distress of difficulty breathing is the only thing keeping someone alive. In such a case, it would be cruel to deprive someone of relief only to make them suffer longer. And also, one must remember, it is the disease that is killing the patient, not the medication. There should be no guilt in giving the last dose of comfort to a dying patient. There will always be a last dose of medicine given. Families have been frightened about giving the dose and the patient dying. A daughter was once very distraught because she had given her mother morphine and the patient died within minutes. In that length of time, minimal medication would have gotten into the patient's system so the drug could not have caused her death. It was simply her time.

Last Gift

Elena knew her brother Nicolae was very sick and on hospice in the United States. She wanted to see him before he died, but living in Romania and being the sole breadwinner for her family did not allow her much time to be away from home. She was in frequent contact with the hospice team to monitor his situation so, if possible, she could come out to see him once more before he died.

But, as can sometimes happen, death can come without warning. Although he was expected to live a few more weeks, Nicolae quietly passed away in his sleep one night. The social worker called Elena to express our condolences and regrets for not being able to give her time to come out.

"Hello, Elena, this is Sara from hospice."

Before Sara could say another word, Elena said, "Nicolae died early this morning, didn't he?"

"Yes," said Sara. "Did someone already call you?"

"No," Elena said. "Nicolae came to me in a dream this morning and said not to worry about him anymore, that he was OK. I knew what he meant, and I am grateful for the help you gave him. It meant a lot to both of us. Nicolae was always the one to worry about me. I think he knew the hardship it would be on me and my family to fly to the United States. This was his last gift to me. Thank you and God bless you for the work you do."

7

MANAGING AGITATION AND DELIRIUM

Problem behavior may occur with any illness and can be a source of great distress and difficulty for family and caregivers. This is frequently seen in dementia patients such as those with Alzheimer's disease but may occur in other patients as well. Dementia patients may often misinterpret their surroundings, who is caring for them, and what the intentions of the caregivers are. Furthermore, they may neither be able to identify the cause of their distress nor express their needs even if they do know what is wrong. Delirium on the other hand can occur in dementia patients or patients who have been cognitively intact. Delirium has many causes, which will be discussed below. The features of this phenomenon include a fluctuating level of consciousness (alert or agitated alternating with lethargy or unresponsiveness). Pulse, blood pressure and temperature may fluctuate, and there may be hallucinations (usually visual). Disorientation or confusion can accompany these other symptoms as well. When problem behaviors occur, there is always a reason for it.

"Agitation" is simply unwanted behavior and not a diagnosis, nor is there a single drug to treat it. It is far better to treat the cause of the behavior than to just impair the patient's ability to express their distress with sedative drugs. A thorough assessment of the patient and a detailed description of the behavior is necessary to resolve the issue. Most of the time this can be done without antipsychotic medication such as haloperidol (Haldol) or Seroquel (quetiapine), both of which carry an FDA Black Box Warning not to give to elderly dementia patients due to increased risk of stroke and death. For example, one of my patients did not respond to Haldol but did respond to removing the thumbtack that was sticking through the bottom of his slipper!

When looking for the cause of unwanted behavior, ask the following questions. Is the patient too hot or too cold? Hungry or thirsty? Is the patient wet or soiled? Is it too bright or too dark? Too crowded or too lonely? Overstimulated or too bored? Too noisy or too quiet? Are glasses or hearing aids missing? Is there constipation or a urinary blockage? Is the patient ill? Is the patient in pain? Was the patient given a new drug such as one with anticholinergic (AC) side effects or even an antibiotic (for example, Cipro can cause delirium)? Has there been a change of location or care givers now unfamiliar to the patient? Check the patient's temperature, feel for a distended bladder, check for impaction. If you still can't resolve the situation, contact the hospice nurse for advice or even a visit.

We received a call one morning from a distraught daughter who had just gotten off the phone with her father who was a hospice patient living alone. She said his conversation was nonsensical, and he seemed to be extremely disoriented and agitated. The hospice nurse and social worker agreed to meet the daughter at the father's house to assess the situation and if necessary, initiate a five-day respite care. It was obvious that the gentleman was confused, agitated, and disoriented. During the course of the visit, the social worker noticed that the glasses he was wearing were not his usual glasses. Also, she noted that she had to speak in a much louder voice for him to hear. The daughter found his correct glasses and the nurse replaced the hearing aid battery and within thirty to forty-five minutes, he was back to his pleasant, capable self. It is scary to think what might have happened if this simple solution had not been found.

Most of the time, if a patient is combative (striking out, scratching, biting, etc.), the problem is pain. Try to identify the cause. If the cause either cannot be determined, or cannot be corrected, treatment for pain should occur prior to the administration of an antipsychotic medication. If pain medication is not helpful, or only partially helpful, medication for anxiety may be effective. Antidepressants like citalopram (Celexa) have been shown to be effective for some patients, not only in managing depression within two to three weeks but also in managing agitation within two to three days. Antidepressants to be avoided are Prozac (fluoxetine) as it can cause anxiety, kill the appetite, and remain in the system a long time after stopping it; also, paroxetine (Paxil) should be avoided as it is the most anticholinergic (AC) of this group of antidepressants. Often distraction with something of interest to the patient or redirection to another activity will help. Calming interventions such as soothing music or lavender oil can help calm the patient as well. The use of an audio or, even better, video, baby monitor can be very helpful in monitoring the safety of the patient when the caregiver needs to be in another room for a while.

I Love You, Mommy

A faulty latch on the swimming pool gate led to tragedy. Two-year-old Joey was found face down in the water. Prolonged efforts to revive him restored his heartbeat, but now it was only the machines in the ICU keeping him alive. His mom, Nicole, had been at his bedside for three days with virtually no sleep. With his vital signs stable, the nurses finally talked her into going home and getting some rest.

At home, she collapsed in bed and finally cried herself to sleep. She dreamed of her little boy. He was walking up to her waving.

"Mommy, I have something to tell you." She heard him say, "I'm OK now. I'm OK, but I have to go. Bye, Mommy. I love you."

She awoke to the telephone ringing. A somber voice on the other end said, "Nicole, this is the hospital. Could you come down here right away?"

Her intuition had already told her what happened. Joey's heart had stopped again, but this time all attempts had failed to restart it. At least she got to say good-bye.

8

PREVENTING FALLS

Falls are the number one cause of accidental death in the elderly. As the frail and elderly have such thin skin and brittle bones, innumerable injuries are caused by falls each year. By taking some simple precautions, many of these falls can be avoided. Hospice patients have enough suffering and limitations without the additional pain and disability that falls can cause.

Let's start with the home environment. Make sure the areas the patient uses have adequate lighting. Natural lighting is best, as it helps the patient maintain normal circadian rhythm (keeping their days and nights straight). Natural daylight helps the patient to stay awake in the daytime and sleep at night. Also, adequate lighting reduces the risk of confusion and disorientation (which are also risks for falls), problems that can occur with any hospice patient. Plenty of light helps the patient to see objects on the floor (toys, cats, spills, etc.) and avoid stepping on them. Highly reflective surfaces such as polished wood or tile floors, or granite countertops, can reflect direct sunlight and be blinding to patients who have cataracts. Translucent window coverings can help with that. Lighting at night should be low but still adequate to allow safe navigation for the patient who can still walk.

Next is the risk of home furnishings. Even slightly uneven flooring, such as where a wood floor transitions to carpet or single steps to sunken dining or living rooms can be hazardous. Low-lying furniture such as coffee tables and ottomans should be removed from the patient's traffic areas. Electrical cords need to be well out of the way. The highest risk object for falls in the home are area rugs. They make the walking surface uneven, especially if they are fringed or the edges are curling. Small rugs on slick floors can slide causing patients to fall.

Many patients are confused at their baseline. Others become confused when it is getting dark ("sundowning"). Still others may transition to a confused state as the disease progresses. Still others may have temporary confusion due to side effects of a medication or at the onset of infection. Weakness or loss of balance may accompany these changes, or the patient simply may not remember that they are unable to walk.

Bed rails may pose as much of a hazard as a help in preventing falls. Half rails do help a weak but clear-headed patient reposition in bed. But a confused patient who tries to climb over the rails will then fall from the height of the rails (not just the height of the mattress). Or the patient may get an arm or leg entangled in the rails during a fall, causing even more severe injury. Tying patients in bed has been abandoned in facilities (and should not be used in the home) because of injuries and even strangulation. Bolstering the patient with pillows on either side may be a compromise measure to keep the patient in bed. If all else fails, placing the mattress on the floor and a pad beside the mattress can be very effective in preventing falls.

Medications that help the patient sleep through the night can be helpful but can also cause confusion and impair balance if the patient awakens before the medications wear off. Your hospice doctor may recommend medication if anxiety, hallucinations, or delusions are contributing to the patient's restlessness. To prevent falls during transfers from bed to wheelchair, hospice can pay for a one-time physical therapy evaluation for instruction in transferring and any needs for additional equipment such as a transfer pole (a vertical pole from floor to ceiling to steady the patient during transfers). Deep recliner chairs (Geri Chairs) may help keep the patient from getting up unassisted as well. As the blood shifts to the intestines after meals, elderly patients are more susceptible to blood pressure dropping when going from a sitting to standing position. After meals the patient should not be rushed to leave the table and should stand for a moment before starting to walk.

There are many medications that can contribute to falls. Medications for pain, anxiety, or sleep as well as muscle relaxants and any of the anticholinergic (AC) class of drugs can cause drowsiness, weakness, or loss of balance. Blood pressure medications may need to be reduced as the patient loses weight, to prevent fainting or dizziness on standing. Water pills for heart, kidney, or liver disease can also drop blood pressure. The risk of falls, as well as the risk for other side effects, is why we review all the patients' medications at least every other week. If dizziness or light-headedness become a problem, the hospice nurse should be contacted right away. Prevention of falls is far better than dealing with the consequences of them.

Hope

As the hospice medical director for the region, I am often asked to meet with "difficult" families who are not willing to cooperate with the hospice staff. The RN case manager asked me to see if I could get better cooperation from the Roberts family who were "quite strange" and were placing unreasonable restrictions on the visits the team members were trying to make.

The case was quite unusual as our patient, Hope, was only twenty-six years old and had been suffering from a poorly defined autoimmune disease that she had since childhood. Any treatment the doctors tried just made her feel worse, and she finally refused any further care and wanted only to be kept comfortable at home where she was now debilitated to the point of being bedbound.

Hope and her family were brilliant, amazingly artistic, and highly educated in the realms of the world religions and were primarily Christian but saw deep spiritual connections to many other religions. They declined chaplain support as they felt they had their need already met in that regard, and they did not want additional visitors. Hope found visitors incredibly difficult to tolerate as touching her caused severe pain and her strength to interact was nearly gone.

It was not just the stressful spiritual energy of the staff in her bedroom that she could not tolerate, she could also sense their presence downstairs in the living room where their inaudible conversations would cause her enormous anxiety. My concerns that she was delusional, or simply manipulative, disappeared when the office got a call during her weekly case review that our current discussion several miles away was causing her distress, and they wanted to know how much longer we would be talking about her.

I couldn't wait to meet them. I too had a strong interest in Christianity, the other world religions, and psychic phenomena. So, when I met them, the family and I really connected, and bridges of trust were built that allowed us to address their bereavement needs and Hope's comfort needs. I had no idea of the amazing depth and talent that Hope possessed. As our relationship grew, they began to share with me her profound poetry and beautiful, intricately detailed art-work of the visions that she had had since she was a very young.

Hope's dad, Robert, would often go for long runs to deal with the stress of watching his beautiful and talented daughter slip away. On one run, when her time was getting near, he was captivated by the beauty of the cherry blossoms on the trees on his run. He stopped, lay down on the grass, and looked up through the delicate flowers at the clear blue sky. Hope, like the flowers, was a gift from God, sweet and beautiful, but given only for a moment in time, to give a glimpse of Heaven. Robert knew then the heartbreak God must feel making the choice to bless us for a brief time with an angel and leave us with the grieve of her departure, or never allow us to see what his loving creative hand can do.

When Robert returned from his run, he went quietly upstairs and kissed Hope on the forehead. She woke up and said, "I saw you in the flowers."

Knowing her far too well to be surprised at anything she said, he asked, "What flowers?"

She smiled weakly, "You were looking up through the flowers thinking of me. Always remember me when you see them."

"Baby girl, I won't need flowers to remember you."

Several days later, Hope shook off the last tentacles that this world of sorrow and suffering had on her. Her family missed her terribly but knew there was rejoicing somewhere else.

I went by to see them a week or so later to check on them.

"I can't imagine how hard it must be, now that she's gone," I comforted.

A smile crept across Robert's face, "She only died. What makes you think she's gone?"

With anyone else that response would be only poetic. Knowing Hope, I could only imagine…

9

MANAGING NAUSEA AND VOMITING

Nausea and vomiting are terrible symptoms to endure and may have many causes. Remember, nausea and vomiting are *symptoms* of another problem, not a single disease with a single treatment. The challenge of managing these daunting symptoms is reduced by addressing the causes of the symptoms, not just covering them up. Nausea and vomiting can be caused, or worsened, by medications, constipation, inner-ear problems, increased pressure on the brain, obstruction of the intestines, chronic disease, new infections, and many other causes. When reporting these symptoms to your doctor or the hospice nurse, the key is to first evaluate the loved one you are caring for. Know their list of diseases, their list of medications, their last bowel movement, their temperature, and any recent changes in other symptoms, before calling.

Medications, medications, medications! Any time anything is wrong with anyone, first think medications. Pain medications of the opiate variety, especially codeine and morphine, can have the direct side effect of vomiting. It's important to remember that just because one or two medications in this class have these, or other, side effects does not mean that all the medications in this class will have the same side effects. Other opiate pain medications may be fine. In addition to their direct effect, constipation caused by these medications may be the reason for loss of appetite, nausea, or vomiting.

New infections (especially bladder infections), and, very commonly, the antibiotics to treat them, can cause nausea and vomiting. One particular condition, labyrinthitis, which is inflammation of the inner ear (the balance center) can cause severe nausea and vomiting. This condition causes a false sensation of moving or spinning called vertigo. It can be caused by medications, infections, or even stroke. Treatment of this is over-the-counter meclizine (Antivert). More severe cases respond to low doses of Valium (diazepam).

Medications that were not previously a problem, such as digoxin, can be a cause because of the toxic levels of the drug when the kidneys can no longer clear it from the body due to dehydration or kidney failure from other causes. Nausea or vomiting can be a problem for many medications in many different classes, for many different reasons. For example, if the patient is diabetic, they may have nerve damage causing difficulty in emptying the stomach into the intestines. If they take something over-the-counter to make them sleep (especially, anything in the

Benadryl class of drugs called anticholinergics—described in earlier chapters), the muscles in the stomach wall may be completely paralyzed, causing a rapid feeling of fullness after eating only a small amount, regurgitation, and vomiting. If nerve damage is the problem, a drug that stimulates the muscles in the stomach lining, such as Reglan (metoclopramide), may help greatly.

The best thing to do is to stop the medication that is, or maybe causing, the problem. If you don't know which drug is to blame, contact the hospice nurse or your physician in order to stop any medications not essential for symptom management. It is certainly wise to stop all vitamins, supplements, and all nonessential over-the-counter medications as they just add to the "pill burden" and increase the risk of choking.

If cancer chemotherapy drugs are still being taken, or recently stopped, or there is any other medication, toxin, or chemical causing the nausea and vomiting (often caused by poor liver or kidney function), vomiting may not relieve the nausea. Medications such as Zofran (ondansetron) or other drugs in this category (antidopaminergic class) works best. This class of drugs specifically targets the part of the brain (the chemoreceptor trigger zone) where chemicals in the blood are causing the vomiting. Because the offending agent is in the blood, not the stomach, vomiting usually does not relieve the nausea.

Nausea characterized by a burning sensation in the upper abdomen, which is lessened by eating, may be gastritis (inflammation of the stomach lining). If the burning sensation is under the breast bone after eating, it is likely to be due to acidic contents of the stomach pushed or leaking up into the lower esophagus (food tube). Smoking, alcohol, caffeine, and fatty or spicy foods may make this worse. These symptoms are usually promptly relieved by antacids such as Rolaids or Tums, and if frequent, by medications that reduce acid production such as Pepcid, Zantac, Prilosec, or Prevacid. These drugs may affect kidney function, so check with the doctor first if the patient has kidney problems.

Cancers are often treated by the body as something foreign, causing inflammation and swelling. When cancer starts (or spreads to) the brain, swelling usually occurs and severe headaches and vomiting result. Steroids such as dexamethasone (Decadron) reduce swelling and inflammation and often can relieve the headaches and vomiting. If a cancer in or around the intestine is causing a blockage, steroids may relieve or reduce the blockage. Steroids are often followed a couple of days later by medication, such as Reglan (metoclopramide), to increase the activity of the bowel, which may have been overstretched by the blockage. Each dexamethasone dose lasts long enough that it need only be given once a day in the morning with food. If the dose is high enough to upset the stomach, the dose can be split between breakfast and lunch. Giving it late in the day can interfere with sleep.

If the blockage is total and does not respond to steroids, injections to stop the production of intestinal fluid (octreotide) can be given to reduce the build-up of fluid and reduce vomiting. If there is a single location in the intestine in a patient who would otherwise have comfortable weeks to months to live, surgical interventions may be considered under hospice care. For a total blockage, tumor removal may be considered, with or without a stoma emptying the bowel into a collection bag.

Partial blockages, if accessible with scopes, may temporarily be relieved with a plastic tube through the narrowed area, to allow the passage of intestinal contents. If intestinal blockage is severe, irreversible and/or extensive, a procedure called "a venting gastrostomy" may be possible by the radiologist. This is a tube that goes through the abdominal wall into the stomach and is attached to suction to remove air and fluid build-up that can trigger vomiting. Even with this device in place, hospice has a number of ways for the family to give medications for pain and other symptom management (under the tongue, rectally, or through the skin by needle or catheter).

If there are many causes for the nausea and vomiting, or the cause is unknown, the medication we find most effective is haloperidol. Compazine/prochlorperazine (which is more sedating and has more side effects) can be given by rectal suppository if needed. For immediate, temporary relief from nausea and vomiting, while waiting for prescription medication to arrive or kick in, a recent article suggested tearing open an alcohol swab and sniffing the vapors released from it. Our limited experience with this measure has been found to be effective.

Rainbow

Theresa was torn as to what she should do. Her mother, Jackie, who lived in Ohio was nearing the end of a losing battle with cancer. But here in California, her son was about to graduate high school, and she was chairing the graduation committee that was in charge of the senior party, the ceremony, and other activities that were at their most critical stage. Her mom was not just her mother, she was also her best friend. The two had a special connection that was hard to explain.

Theresa called her mom to tell her she would drop what she was doing and come out to see her one last time.

"Don't you dare," Jackie told Theresa. "You need to be there for your son. It would break my heart if you let him down. I'll be at the graduation."

"But Mom, you're way too sick to travel. From what Dad tells me, you're not even likely to make it till then." Theresa said, her voice starting to crack with emotion.

"I'll be there. Just look for the rainbow. I love you both so much. Don't worry."

Theresa was a little confused by her mom's reply, but wrote it off to the pain medication she was needing in ever increasing doses. Jackie always loved rainbows ever since her trip to Hawaii and had them decorating many of the things in her house. She could talk to her later when she was clearer.

Two days later at exactly 7:50 p.m., Theresa suddenly knew her mom had died. She didn't know how she knew, but she knew. She waited for her dad to call. An hour later the phone rang. When she answered, she didn't even say hello, "Dad, Mom's gone, isn't she? She died an hour ago."

"Yes, how did you know?" he answered, not entirely surprised, knowing their connection.

"I don't know. I just felt it. Graduation is tomorrow, but I'll fly back to see you day after tomorrow."

Theresa remembered what her mom had said about the rainbow, but fair skies in June in California would keep her away even symbolically.

The next day, graduation went as planned, except for one thing. There was a rare meteorological occurrence called a "sun dog" that day. This is when ice crystals in the upper atmosphere refract a spot of sunlight into…a rainbow fragment. Grandma kept her word.

10

MANAGEMENT AND PREVENTION OF SKIN BREAKDOWN

The skin that covers our bodies is the largest organ of the body and does many amazing things. It is our first line of defense against the world outside. Heat, cold, trauma, infection, toxins, parasites, and damaging radiation all must breach the barrier that covers our entire body. Skin stabilizes our body temperature, prevents dehydration, converts vitamins to their useful form, gives us precisely detailed information about the world outside, and provides some of our greatest pleasures through softness, warmth, touch, and intimacy.

But as the springy elastic fibers in our skin age, they lose their agility to recoil and restore the youthful smoothness and thickness. Skin begins to sag and wrinkle. As skin stretches out with age, it becomes thinner and more fragile. When the skin can no longer stretch when it is pulled, the connections between the skin layers give way and a partial-thickness flap of skin can be pulled off, called a "skin tear." These are common in the elderly and even minor trauma can cause these tears or areas of bruising between layers of the skin. Even pulling a patient up in bed by grabbing the wrist and pulling can cause a tear. Your hospice nurse will be glad to instruct you in safer ways to reposition your loved one.

With hospital beds or other adjustable beds, make sure to put the foot of the bed up when the head of the bed is raised. Just the friction of the skin of the back and buttocks against the sheet can cause skin breakdown from the shearing force of sliding down in the bed. Also, it is much easier to move the patient up in bed if you put the head of the bed down first, slide the patient up, then raise the head of the bed again. Shearing-type skin breakdown is more common if the skin remains moist from sweat or urine. Prolonged contact of skin with a soiled diaper will quickly cause inflammation and breakdown. Moisturizing lotions and barrier creams are very useful in preserving skin integrity.

Patients who are weak, lethargic, or unresponsive from disease or medication do not move much, if at all, on their own. As nutritional and fluid intake decline, muscle and fat are lost and the bony prominences of the skeleton put additional stress on the skin. The pressure of the tailbone, for example, on the thin skin can cut off all circulation to that area of skin. If the patient is not frequently repositioned, that skin will become injured and even die, causing a pressure sore. It is important to reposition patients at least every two hours in order to prevent skin breakdown. A pillow under the calves of the legs "floats" the heels and prevents skin breakdown there.

The first sign of skin damage is when the skin remains red when gentle finger pressure is applied and then removed from the area. Next, the surface of the skin begins to break down. The wound may extend completely through the skin into the fat layer below the skin. If the pressure is not relieved, the wound can extend deep into the muscle layers and down to the bone. Frequent repositioning is necessary to prevent this.

However, in the last few days, when death is imminent, over-attention to skin care may cause more pain and suffering than leaving the patient in their most comfortable position. In this situation, skin breakdown may be inevitable. What is hard for caregivers to grasp is that the most important thing is insuring the dying patient's comfort, even when it results in skin breakdown. In the last days of life, turning the patient should only be for cleaning and comfort, not for prevention of skin breakdown. Maintaining pristine skin, at the cost of increased suffering, is not consistent with the hospice philosophy of putting the comfort of the patient first.

As pressure wounds are caused by (you guessed it) pressure, the key to prevention and healing is elimination, or at least reduction, of pressure. Adequate nutrition and hydration are also important in healing, but in hospice patients that always becomes a losing battle. Dead tissue within the wounds is usually managed with creams that dissolve protein. Large amounts of dead tissue, or large, hard platelike scabs may need to be removed with surgical instruments.

If the wound is producing a lot of drainage or odor, a powdered form of antibiotic (usually metronidazole/

Flagyl) can be sprinkled directly on the wound. Most large wounds have no chance of healing in the time frame of the hospice patient. For this reason, we often use Betadine-soaked gauze to keep odor and drainage in check. We do not use this treatment in wounds we believe can resolve as the iodine solution slows healing. Oral antibiotics have no place in healing pressure wounds, unless the healthy tissue around the wound is showing signs of deep-tissue infection (called cellulitis). In addition, oral antibiotics can cause nausea and loss of appetite, and often diarrhea, which not only worsens diaper area wounds but increases the patient's discomfort with the required increase in changing and cleaning. Finally, getting a culture of the surface of the wound is useless, as the results would not reliably tell us what bacteria is causing the infection.

Hospice nurses and physicians are usually adequately trained in the management of pressure wounds. Many hospice organizations have specially trained wound nurses or access to physicians who specialize in wound management. But again, specialized aggressive wound management has a limited place in hospice, where the wounds are not likely to heal in the time the patient has left. Management of symptoms remains the top priority. Prevention of wound formation or worsening, and control of pain, odor, and drainage will preserve the patient's comfort and dignity, as well as the family's peace of mind.

He's Gone

Bill and Dorothy had been married for sixty-eight wonderful years. Now they were both on hospice, sharing a room in a board and care. Della, the hospice nurse, visited them every week. Dorothy was bedbound with Alzheimer's disease, and Bill was tethered by a green tube to his oxygen concentrator and barely able to get himself to his recliner chair only three steps away. His heart was failing fast. Dorothy had always been a chatterbox. She was constantly talking to him every waking moment. Unfortunately, as her memory slipped away, her depression and anxiety grew. Her usual pleasant banter was gradually replaced with fretfulness and calling out for Bill day and night.

Seeing her sinking into the cruel clutches of dementia, and unable to console her cries for help, was an unbearable burden on Bill's fragile heart. To make matters worse, Lenora, the facility director, said Dorothy was becoming too disruptive for her facility and she would have to be moved to a nursing home several miles away. The separation literally broke Bill's heart. Now, with Dorothy gone, Bill rapidly declined. Within weeks, his heart finally gave out and he passed away. Because of fears that Dorothy would become even more agitated if told of Bill's death, Lenora asked Della not to tell Dorothy of his passing.

Since moving to the nursing home, Dorothy continued her mental decline. Despite their separation, she continued to chatter to Bill as if she were still in her room at the board and care and call out to him day and night. But when Della came by to see Dorothy about a week after Bill died, Dorothy was quiet and had been so for the past few days according to staff.

Della took her hand and asked cautiously, "Dorothy, why aren't you talking to Bill?"

"He's gone." Dorothy said quietly. "He came to say good-bye and that he would see me soon."

The next day, they were together again. But this time forever.

11

MANAGING SLEEP

Families and caregivers are probably hoping that this chapter is for them. Caring for a dying loved one is not just heartbreaking, it is also exhausting. If the patient can get on the right sleep schedule, that will go a long way to helping the family and caregivers to get the sleep that they need to continue to do their labor of love. So indirectly this chapter is for them as well.

Managing the sleep cycles of demented or dying patients is often a great challenge. There are interventions that can improve the situation of a patient who is up all night and sleeps all day, other than moving to Singapore and hoping the time change will solve everything. First, assess the *patient* for anything that might be keeping them awake during the nighttime hours. Second, assess the *environment* for things that are aggravating the problem. Third, try some *interventions* that may help.

Please refer to chapter 7 for the management of agitation and delirium. Also, it is important to understand sleep patterns in the elderly. Many elderly folks require less sleep, often only about six hours a night. This means that if you put Grandpa to bed at 7:00 p.m., he will have had a full night's sleep by 1:00 a.m. Also, if Grandpa sleeps during the day, he will need less sleep at night. Keeping him awake during the day and up until 10:00 p.m. or 11:00 p.m. with the rest of the family may work out better. Make sure the patient has as little pain, discomfort, and distress as possible. When distraction and stimulation with noise, activity, and light are gone, perception of pain may be increased. If the patient takes pain medication during the day, it would be wise to make sure that it is also given before bed.

Depression and anxiety may be big problems in allowing the patient to get to sleep or stay asleep. Depression is usually more of a problem early in the hospice course and usually in patients who are mentally intact. Sleep disturbance with depression is usually early morning wakening. Patients wake up at 3:00 a.m. or 4:00 a.m. and ruminate over financial or other issues. Asking the patient if he is depressed is usually a sensitive and reliable indicator of a problem. With anxiety, the patient usually has problems going to sleep.

Make sure you ask about thoughts of suicide. Suicidal people are generally more likely than not to admit to such thoughts. If they are having thoughts of suicide, ask if they have a plan. Elderly white males are the highest suicide risk group. Men tend to end their lives in a more violent manner and are more often successful in suicide attempts compared to women. Women are more likely to overdose on medication. There is significant overlap, so if the patient is having suicidal thoughts, lock up all firearms or remove them from the home. Secure prescription medications in a locked box or cabinet. Contact the hospice nurse or the patient's physician for medication for depression as soon as possible. The hospice chaplain or social worker may be very helpful in counseling the patient and helping them work through these tough life issues.

Environmental issues may be key factors in interfering with adequate sleep. Often, when I do home visits, I will walk in the house on a bright sunny day, into the gloom of a living room that has all the curtains shut, a single 25-watt-bulb table lamp, and the patient dozing in the recliner chair in front of the TV where they spend twenty-four hours a day. Humans are designed to be awake during the day and sleep at night. We have a circadian rhythm that keeps us on our day/night schedule. Depriving ourselves of that rhythm will interfere with our cognitive efficiency during the day and our sleep at night.

Making sure there is adequate natural light during the day with mental and physical stimulation will make the patient more prepared for sleep at night. Keeping the curtains open during the day and keeping a regular schedule of bedtime and awakening will maximize sleep cycle success. Melatonin at night may help when starting this program.

Limiting caffeine, alcohol and fluids in the evening will also help. Caffeine may increase anxiety and make it harder to go to sleep. Alcohol may have a rebound effect, waking the patient up when it wears off in the middle of the night. Fluids may require more bathroom trips, especially in men with prostate issues. Unless the patient has a bladder catheter, do not give diuretics (water pills) at night. If they are prescribed twice daily, it is fine to take them morning and noon.

For the maximum chance of sleep at night, make sure the room is much darker and quieter than during the day. If the patient can get out of bed unassisted, make sure there is enough light to navigate to the bathroom. Also, make sure the floor is clear of clutter, spills, cords, and area rugs, all of which can cause tripping risks. If noise outside or inside may wake the patient up, use a white-noise generator (baby-supply stores have them).

Lavender essential oil can be relaxing. Over-the-counter sleep aids that are less likely to cause trouble are chamomile, tryptophan, valerian root, kava-kava, and melatonin. Avoid the older antihistamine-type sleep aids (Benadryl, diphenhydramine, anything PM, etc.).

Prescription drugs you can speak with your physician about are the antidepressant types (Remeron, trazadone, Silenor, and others). Avoid the tricyclics such as amitriptyline/Elavil, etc. Other sleep medications like Ambien/zolpidem, temazepam, and Restoril are good for short-term or occasional use, but they lose their effectiveness over time.

Sleep management may be a complex and difficult problem to deal with. There may be many factors in play, but by carefully assessing the patient for correctable problems, avoiding things that are exacerbating the problem, and introducing interventions to treat the problem, there can be hope for a better situation. If all else fails, and collapse of the caregiver network starts to risk the health of the patient or caregivers, remember that with hospice there is a respite benefit that can allow the patient to be cared for in a contracted facility for up to five days, in order to provide a break for the caregivers and allow time for the hospice team to modify the plan of care so that the patient may return home to live out their days in comfort.

Not Yet, Sister

Lorna was in the late stages of Alzheimer's disease. For months she was mute and bedbound. The caregivers at her facility were trying to feed her, but she took in very little. Her children knew her time was not long, so they were making more frequent visits to make sure Mom was comfortable as her life was slowly ebbing away.

But one day when they visited, they were shocked by the sound coming from their mother's room. It was half of a conversation, as if someone were talking on the phone. But what was so surprising was that it was their mother's voice—a clear, strong voice they had not heard for months.

"No, Ellie, I can't. I'm not ready yet. I'll be there soon, dear. Don't worry about me."

Lorna's conversation ended abruptly as soon as the surprised children walked in the room, expecting their mother had experienced some kind of miraculous recovery. But as they approached the bed, they were met with the silence and the same blank stare they had seen for months. After giving her kisses and a few loving comments, they dejectedly left her alone in bed.

The next morning the phone rang. It was a cousin from New York.

"Hi, guys. I just wanted to let you know that Aunt Ellie died yesterday."

12

MANAGING BLEEDING

The symptom that is often the most alarming to families and caregivers is bleeding. Everything in our DNA tells us to panic at the sight of that crimson warning that something is terribly wrong. Much of the time, bleeding is unexpected and needs to be stopped. At other times, it is a predictable and ongoing problem to be managed. Still in other situations, it is a welcomed sign that the patient's suffering is going to come to a gentle, quiet, and painless end.

Bleeding caused by trauma is almost always a situation requiring first aid to stop the loss of blood. The bleeding can occur underneath the skin as bruising (sometimes very extensive). Or if the bleeding is no longer confined to the body, it easily makes itself known. In the vast majority of cases, the RICE protocol (rest, immobilization, compression, and elevation) will manage things until help can be obtained. Ice is helpful to reduce the extension of bleeding under the skin, such as with sprains, fractures, contusions (blunt trauma), or bumps on the head ("goose-eggs").

Bleeding can also be caused by disease such as inherited clotting disorders, leukemia, deficiencies or malfunction of platelets in the blood, severe vitamin C deficiency, spontaneous rupture of weakened blood vessels, fragile cancers that erupt through the skin, airways, or GI tract, or acquired diseases interfering with the normal production of clotting factors such as liver disease. Medications that interfere with blood clotting (aspirin, anti-inflammatories, antidepressants, and others), may cause or worsen bleeding. Medications that irritate the lining of the stomach such as steroids or anti-inflammatories can cause ulcers and stomach bleeding. Avoiding problem medications, if possible, or mitigating the risks with acid-blocking medications is usually advised.

Situations with difficult-to-control bleeding can occur in the hospice setting, requiring particular management to avoid the difficult and painful transport of patients to the emergency room. For example, when breast cancers, head or neck cancers, or other cancers erode through the skin, they may cause continuous oozing of blood from their raw surfaces, which can be quite extensive if they are large. This occurs most often at dressing changes when bandages can stick to the open areas. If the bleeding is more severe than usual, you may need to buy some time while the hospice nurse is on the way out to evaluate the situation. This is often easily and effectively done with the application of a long-acting decongestant nasal spray (such as Afrin) to the bleeding surface. This type of medication causes powerful constriction of the blood vessels, which may markedly reduce the bleeding.

Nose bleeds can often be very difficult to control. Most nosebleeds are anterior, that is, coming from the flexible cartilage portion of the nose, that is the wall between the two sides, extending out beyond the nasal bones. Elevating the head of the bed and pinching the nose shut with the thumb on one side of the cartilage and the index finger on the other will often stop the bleeding. If after ten minutes or so this doesn't work, placing a damp tea bag in the side that is bleeding and reapplying pressure may help greatly. Black teas have a chemical in them that works topically to cauterize the bleeding surface. If the nasal passages are too small for a whole tea bag, Lipton makes flow-through double bags that are half the size and can be separated with scissors. Moist tea bags can also be used for dental socket or other mucous membrane oozing of blood.

The sight of blood is alarming, especially with large quantities. Such bleeding may be inevitable, such as with uterine, GI, or head and neck cancers. Despite the distressing appearance, dying from blood loss may be a quick and merciful escape from the severe and challenging suffering the disease may be causing. If a large amount of blood loss is an expected risk, it is best to be prepared by using dark-colored sheets on the bed and having an abundant supply of dark towels. There are some medications that can reduce bleeding, such as AMICAR (aminocaproic acid). This medication has been shown to be very useful in reducing bleeding from bladder and prostate cancers in patients who have a good quality of life and still some time to live. However, in those facing death in the next couple of weeks or less, it can cause blood clots, strokes, and other severe side effects while simply prolonging the inevitable. If profuse bleeding is so distressing that the family can no longer care for the patient, the patient may be admitted to the hospital or a skilled nursing facility under the "general inpatient" hospice benefit, until the situation can be managed with a plan of care that can be duplicated at home.

The Hummingbird

Albert was ninety-eight years old and at the very end stages of Alzheimer's disease. He and Margaret had been married for sixty-nine years, most of them in the same small house near Sacramento. Albert had to be moved to a small board-and-care facility in a beautiful rural area near Folsom Lake, east of Sacramento, since Margaret was taken to the hospital. Margaret had recently suffered a heart attack, and after a lengthy hospital stay, she had been transferred to a skilled nursing facility in a nearby suburb for an attempt at rehab. Prior to her hospitalization, despite her frailty, she had been Albert's primary care giver. Without her at his side, Albert quickly began to decline.

Margaret was the light of Albert's life. She had decorated their home of many years with designs of her favorite creatures, hummingbirds. There were hummingbird photos, drawings, and paintings. Glass and ceramic hummingbirds adorned every window sill and shelf. There were even hummingbirds on her dish towels. She also had hummingbird feeders outside the windows of her kitchen and bedroom.

Margaret did not improve. On Sunday, she passed away quietly and alone in her room in rehab. Their daughter Sharon visited Albert the next day but did not tell him what had happened with Margaret. He was too advanced in his disease to be able to understand, let alone remember anything she said for more than a minute or two. But today Albert was restless and agitated. He kept reaching out, grasping for something in the air. Albert had been blind for years, so Sharon thought he must be hallucinating, which she had recently learned was not uncommon with Alzheimer's patients at the end of life.

"What are you reaching for, Dad?" Sharon asked.

"Your mother. Your mother," Albert whispered.

"How long has he been doing this?" Sharon asked the aid who had just walked into the room.

"Since yesterday. About the same time that hummingbird at the window there has kept trying to get in." she said.

Sharon turned and looked toward the window. She was stunned to see a beautiful little hummingbird that kept hovering just outside, frequently bouncing off the glass, but she said nothing.

That night, Albert passed away, and the hummingbird was not seen again.

Sharon came the next day to pick up Albert's belongings.

"Strangest thing. That little hummingbird was trying to get to Albert, and now they're both gone!" the aid mentioned. "Strangest thing!"

Sharon just smiled. "Not strange at all," she thought, "not strange at all."

13

MEDICATIONS

As the end approaches, medications other than for comfort have a rapidly diminishing role in hospice care. As the body is shutting down, the ability of the liver and kidneys to clear medication from the body diminishes, and blood levels may start to rise despite no change in dosage. Medications that are distributed throughout the water in the body also show increased blood levels as dehydration sets in. Medication that was, in large degree, inactive as it was bound to the proteins in the blood have a stronger effect when those protein levels drop due to inadequate nutrition or inadequate absorption of adequate intake. The same blood levels have more of the active unbound form of the drug. These and many other factors increase the side effects and drug interactions of medications that the patient may have been taking for years without problems.

Cholesterol medications have no place in hospice care. Not only is their benefit for years down the road far longer than the hospice patient's expected survival time, but these medications can cause additional muscle pain and weakness in patients whose main problems are already discomfort and debility.

Similarly, diabetic medications are adjusted to keep blood-sugar levels where they will not cause organ damage years later. As oral intake for hospice patients usually declines, the problem for diabetics becomes one of low blood sugar with weakness, sweating, confusion, fainting, and seizures. Symptoms from very high blood-sugar levels mainly include thirst, increased urination, and blurry vision. These symptoms are usually seen at blood sugar levels above five hundred. In hospice we set a target blood sugar range of two hundred to three hundred and fifty, as this range cannot cause trouble for years. As the end approaches, and patients cannot take their oral medications, we recommend no longer checking blood sugar levels, unless we are suspecting high or low levels to be the cause of symptoms that we cannot treat in other ways than blood-sugar control.

As body mass decreases and disease progresses, the patient's blood pressure usually drops as well. Tapering these medications prevents fainting or dizziness and falls from low blood pressure on standing. As a patient's discomfort increases with advancing disease, such as cancer, tapering the patient off cardiac medications prevents artificially prolonging suffering when the body is trying to shut down. A cardiac death is infinitely easier, quicker, and more comfortable than most cancer deaths. Heart medications such as diuretics are continued as long as they ease breathing or other symptoms. As oral intake declines, the role of diuretics usually disappears. It makes no sense to force Lasix into a patient who is dehydrated with no edema. At the end of a long illness, a dehydrated patient may continue to have edema in areas that gravity draws body fluids because of to low protein levels. This edema does not respond well to diuretics (water pills).

One exception to our crusade against non-comfort medications is thyroid-replacement medication. Levothyroxine is less considered a medication and more considered a way to restore normal thyroid hormone levels. Low levels of thyroid can result in lethargy, depression, and feeling cold all the time. Replacement of this hormone can lift the mood, give more energy and engagement in social activities, help the patient be able to do more self-care as well as reduce caregiver burden. It lasts for weeks in the system, so it continues to work after the patient can no longer take medications. When swallowing is an issue, it can be stopped four to five weeks before death without the patient experiencing the symptoms of hypothyroidism low (low thyroid hormone levels.).

If a patient is early in their course in hospice and wish to be restored to their current comfortable level of functioning, the use of antibiotics is completely justifiable. As the terminal disease progresses, antibiotics are limited to those infections that are the source of the patient's greatest discomfort. Near the end, antibiotics have no place, as the body uses infections (usually respiratory or urinary) to hasten the end of suffering from such diseases as cancers, respiratory failure, and neurodegenerative disorders.

Multivitamins, in general, provide tremendous benefits but only for the people who *sell* them, especially if they have kids in private colleges or they need a new German car. Nutritional supplements have not been shown to prolong life or increase lean body mass. The same can be said for probiotics. Unless the patient has a condition that has reduced normal intestinal flora, probiotics are just another expense for just another pill that the weakened patient has to try get down with all their other pills.

No appetite stimulant has been shown to prolong life or increase lean body mass. Any weight gain tends to be fat and fluid retention. Steroids, antidepressants, and (possibly) cannabinoids may enhance mood as well as the pleasure of eating, but that is where their benefit ends. Expensive nutritional supplements (Ensure, Boost, etc.) are also a waste of money. A steak-and-potato type diet does just as well, if not better, to gain or maintain weight. Milkshakes are also much tastier and cheaper.

The general consensus on Alzheimer's drugs is that any benefit is modest, temporary, and associated with significant side effects. Aricept is an appetite killer. If the patient has been on any of these for twelve to eighteen months, or has weight loss, the medications should be tapered and stopped. If a dramatic worsening of symptoms occurs, a trial of restarting the medications is reasonable to see if stopping the medications was the cause. One study did demonstrate an improvement on memory testing but did not show that this translated to any reduction in caregiver burden. Nor do these drugs alter the course of the illness or prolong life. As far as over-the-counter brain supplements go, the US government is suing the makers of the expensive and probably useless drug Prevagen for fraud.

Prescription medications are only available by prescription because they are dangerous. The benefits must be well worth the risks, or they should not be taken. As people age, they take more medications and their bodies have a harder time handling them. An additional problem with hospice drugs is the abuse and diversion risk. Controlled drugs should be handled the same way you would handle cash. Would you leave a roll of $100 bills in your medicine cabinet in the hallway bathroom, or worse yet, on the coffee table? Controlled medications should be kept out of sight or better yet locked up.

The Black Butterfly

One of our administrative nurses, Cleo, read a few of these stories and asked to speak to me and related this story:

"Dr. Nesbitt, it is so interesting that the experiences of patients at the end of life are so similar around the world," she commented shyly.

"What do you mean?" I asked.

"Would you like to hear a story about a black butterfly? I'm not sure I want to tell it because I am not superstitious anymore and I don't want to sound crazy."

"I would love to hear it!" I said.

"Well, I grew up in the Philippines in a rural area. My mom had asthma but was doing all right with it. She was only fifty-three. Then one day she said that her father was coming for her. My grandfather had died before I was born and never knew him.

"I asked her what she was talking about, and she pointed out the door to the garden and said, 'See the black butterfly? That is him; he is coming to take me.' I had never seen a black butterfly before and doubted I would know what she was pointing at as all our butterflies are very small. But hovering in the air in one place was a huge, completely black butterfly, many times the size of the others.

"I didn't understand what she meant. I thought it was just some kind of weird joke and dismissed it.

"The next day, my mom got a very bad asthma attack and died. It was quite a shock to everyone as she had been doing so well and had not been sick up to this point," she said solemnly.

After Cleo finished her story, I immediately went to the computer and Googled "Philippines black butterfly." It turns out there is indeed a species of large black butterflies there that are fairly rare. It also said there is a cultural belief that if one comes to you, that you will die soon.

I showed this to her and asked, "Did you know this about black butterflies?"

"No. I had never heard that. In the rural area we lived, there are a lot of things like that which people say that I avoid as they are just superstitions...aren't they?"

14

TUBE FEEDING

A frequent question we are asked when oral intake is dropping off is whether or not some kind of artificial fluids or nutrition can be instituted and if it is covered by hospice. This is a complicated question, and it can only be answered on a case-by-case basis. There are some people who come to hospice after years on tube feeding, for example, from a stroke. Others had a feeding tube placed during their current hospitalization. There are some who have been battling a pelvic or abdominal cancer and are on total nutrition and fluid by IV as their intestines are completely blocked. Some have months to live, but an infection such as pneumonia has them temporarily too weak to take in enough to keep them going. Some insidious neurological diseases leave the mind intact but the body so weak that oral feeding can take several hours per meal.

If we get a patient with a longstanding stroke that has left them without the ability to swallow safely, and a feeding tube was place years ago, or a developmentally disabled patient who has had a feeding tube since birth, hospice pays for it if Medicare or Medicaid has been covering it up to this point. However, if a patient has had a massive stroke or head injury, leaving them totally unresponsive, we have a discussion with the family regarding the goals of care.

Patients who have suffered for months or years with a stroke and are fed with a feeding tube continue to decline despite interventions. The tube-feeding formula inevitably works its way back up the esophagus and into the unprotected windpipe (trachea). This not only causes chemical inflammation in the lungs but also bacterial infections from germs carried by the formula or from oral secretions. These infections become more and more frequent until even antibiotics are of no use. As the body tries to shut down despite aggressive interventions, much of the nutrition poured into the stomach is not absorbed. Muscles waste away, and skin breaks down causing painful pressure sores.

As the patient moves less and less, the nutritional needs can be as little as five hundred calories a day. Higher volumes of formula cause increased choking on fluid (aspiration). A stroke, disease, or injury that destroys the ability to swallow is a fatal one. It is just a matter of time. Aggressive interventions, such as feeding tubes, artificially extend life, but with time the benefits are outweighed by the burden that these measures impose.

As death approaches, despite interventions, patients sleep more and more of the day and lose weight despite adequate caloric replacement. By gradually tapering feedings and flushes, while at the same time observing for any discomfort, and managing any symptoms with comfort medications, the body becomes free to comfortably and peacefully shut down without the suffering caused by interference with this most natural of processes, dying. It is heartbreaking for us in hospice when we see family members allow their guilt and indecision prolong the suffering of a patient who is desperately trying to escape their expended physical shell.

Strokes by their nature bring a sudden loss of the ability to swallow, but with other neurological disorders the process is more gradual. Alzheimer's disease is one where increasing trouble swallowing can be quite frustrating for caregivers and anxiety provoking for families. Diet modification is necessary when increased difficulty swallowing is evidenced by increasing coughing with eating or drinking. Thin liquids and mixed textured foods (such as cold breakfast cereals) seem to give the greatest trouble.

Powders are available to add to liquids to thicken them. Diets can be downgraded from regular to mechanical soft, to chopped, to chopped with sauces and gravies, to pureed. Liquids can be downgraded to nectar thick, honey thick, and finally pudding thick. As a patient approaches the very end of life, they should be allowed to eat whatever foods they like. Usually the last thing they refuse is ice cream. This is not a time to worry about their cholesterol or torture them with a kale and eggplant smoothie.

Feeding tubes are not appropriate for late-stage Alzheimer's patients. The statistics show that they live an average of six months longer with slow spoon feeding than with feeding tubes. Tube-fed Alzheimer's patients get aspiration pneumonia and pressure sores more often. Studies of patients with advanced Alzheimer's disease show they receive no benefit from tube feeding and are at increased risk for complications. Early stage Alzheimer's patients who have temporary swallowing problems or swallowing problems from a blockage may be the exceptions to the rule.

Patients with Lou Gehrig's disease (ALS) may be able to maintain their cognitive abilities long after their strength to feed themselves is gone. Although they may be able to safely swallow, it may take up to four hours to finish a meal. This may become untenable for caregivers. In these patients the placement of a feeding tube may make the difference of whether or not a patient can remain in their home. In this situation hospice may pay for the procedure. The other situation where hospice may pay for a feeding tube placement through the abdominal wall is when the patient may have months to live otherwise but has an obstruction preventing oral feeding such as a head, neck, or esophageal cancer.

We frequently are referred patients with abdominal or pelvic cancers who have complete intestinal blockages requiring all fluids and nutrition to be given IV. Such patients usually only have weeks or less to live. A question that I am frequently asked by these patients is, "How long can I get IV feedings on hospice?" My response is, "As long as you want." I then explain how the fluids and feeding may bring some comfort now, but soon they will become a source of discomfort. In addition, as the cancer is the most metabolically active tissue in the body, artificial nutrition may enhance the growth and spread of the tumor as it steals all the calories we give and still consumes the body tissues as well.

The same is true for patients with poor oral intake who get outpatient IV fluids on a regular basis. On hospice, we tell them, we give IV fluids based on what the patient says, not on what the calendar says. If a patient is becoming uncomfortable from dehydration, we may give IV fluids at that time. If fluids make the patient feel better, function better, and decreases caregiver burden, then it is hospice appropriate to do so.

There are many problems caused by artificial fluids and nutrition in addition to the above-mentioned problems. As the body moves toward death, protein production begins to drop off. One of the proteins is albumen. It is produced by the liver and does many things such as binding with medications and acting as a sponge, holding water inside the blood vessels. When albumen levels are low, the water in the blood vessels seeps into the outside tissues. This resulting fluid accumulation is called "edema."

When this fluid seeps into the brain tissue, it can cause headaches, visual disturbances, problems with cognition, and pressure on the brainstem, which controls the body's vital signs. Fluid seeping into the lung tissue interferes with oxygen transfer into the blood and can obstruct the airways causing severe shortness of breath. Fluid seeping into the intestinal walls causes bowel wall edema and poor peristalsis (bowel movement) with resultant decreased bowel movement and perhaps bowel distention and discomfort. As the kidneys try to excrete the extra fluids, more urine production also results in more frequent turning, cleaning, and changing. The extra bladder and bowel output also irritate the skin and increase the risk of breakdown. Large fluid collections in the tissues in bedbound patients result in in swelling, discomfort, and increased difficulty moving.

But what may cause the most suffering from forcing fluids and nutrition into dying patients is the interference with the body's natural process of shutting down. Because feeding someone is the most fundamental human display of love, families often vocalize concerns that *not* giving artificial fluid and nutrition is causing their loved one to die of hunger or thirst. Dying patients *lose* their hunger and *lose* their thirst. You cannot die of something you do not have. It may be culturally important for the patient to receive artificial nutrition or to die with a full stomach, which may require the use of a feeding tube. It is important to respect these cultural concerns.

As the body begins to reject food, it begins to breakdown fat. This causes the breakdown products of fat (ketones) to accumulate in the blood. This results in a sense of euphoria and spiritual clarity, preparing the patient for transition from this life. This state of high ketones in the blood, or ketosis, is also the result of fasting, which is a spiritual discipline of most of the world's religions.

As fluid intake tapers off, there is a build-up of the breakdown products of proteins in the blood, called urea. Urea is usually flushed out of the body into the urine (from the term urea) by the intake of fluid. Urea is an amazing chemical for the dying patient as it relieves suffering in many ways. First, it relieves pain. Second, it relieves anxiety. Third, it peacefully and comfortably puts the patient into a final deep sleep to ease the "letting-go" from this life.

Forcing calories into the body deprives it of the euphoria and spiritual clarity of ketosis. Forcing fluids into the body flushes out the comforting and soothing urea that cushions death's final blow. Again, interfering with the body's process of shutting down not only increases suffering but also prolongs it by drawing out the dying process. At hospice we try to work with the body rather than against it. And that makes all the difference in the world.

The Yellow Bird

A very good friend of mine, whom I will call Ryan, is one of the top leaders in a well-known international Christian youth organization. He was at one of their camps, high in the Rocky Mountains, when word was released that the very elderly founder of the organization had died after a brief illness. Word of the leader's death got to Ryan when he and his friend Bob were working out in the gym at the camp. It was heartbreaking for the both of them, and they sat down to console each other as they fought back their tears for their dear friend, mentor, and leader.

As they were talking, they were distracted a very brightly colored yellow bird outside the window. The bird just perched on the back of a chair staring at them through the window and after a few minutes, flew off.

"That's odd," said Ryan. "I've been coming here for fifteen years, and I've never seen a bird like that before."

"Wow! Me neither; it's beautiful," Bob replied. "It must be someone's pet that got loose. We better ask around."

They made the announcement of the unusual bird at dinner, but no one knew where it had come from or had ever seen one in the wild up there before.

A few months later, Bob and Ryan were in Costa Rica helping to start clubs in the inner cities for the youth there. There was great enthusiasm for the project, and they were able to attract crowds of people to hear their message. Shortly after the evening meeting, an elderly local gentleman approached them to thank them for coming and for their wonderful work in the city.

As he was turning to leave, the old man said, "Oh yes, I'm so sorry about your friend."

Bob was puzzled. "I'm sorry, what friend are you talking about?"

"You know, the one in Colorado." He said in a hushed voice, "I was the yellow bird."

Bob and Ryan's jaws dropped as they stared at each other in disbelief. They turned back to ask the old man what he meant, but he had disappeared into the crowd in the gathering darkness and was not seen again.

15

KNOWING THE END IS NEAR

How do you know when the end is approaching? Are there signs that alert you to call the distant relatives? Yes, there are a few. However, not everyone cooperates, even at death's door. In terms of arranging for final family visits, the sooner, the better is the best plan. Often, we see patients abruptly decline or suddenly die much sooner than expected. Having the family visit while the patient is still able to communicate is helpful in creating lasting memories and allowing opportunities for closure. All patients are different in their physiology, state of underlying fitness, and constellation of other diseases that they may have. Every terminal illness is variable in its course. Due to these factors it can be quite challenging to narrow the window in which the patient may die.

As space would not allow for tracking each and every terminal illness, I will address the general principles that we follow in hospice. The first signs that may be seen are increasing weakness and fatigue. This will result in decreasing function, decreasing self-care, and increasing caregiver burden. The patient is likely to start sleeping more and eating less. Weight loss is common, even when oral intake is adequate. As decline continues, the patient becomes bedbound, total care, stops eating, stops drinking, and sleeps almost all the time.

Patients who are nearing the end of life, depending on dozens of other factors, can go about three minutes without breathing, three days without drinking, and three weeks without eating before they die. But just so you know, I pronounced a patient dead after five minutes of no respirations or pulse, who then resumed breathing and lived for about another two hours. Patients with edema (fluid retention) have gone for a week or more without oral intake. Patients taking only sips of fluids (depending on how much and what is in them) have survived several weeks. Food intake diminishes, and the bowels shut down first. Then urine output declines and stops when fluid intake stops and the body's fluid stores are depleted.

Death can come at once if the brain is turned off suddenly due to a heart attack or irregular heart rhythm. More often we see things progress more slowly over time with the patient sleeping more and more and taking in less and less. Brain function begins to shut down due to inefficient breathing, the liver and kidneys failing, and urea, bilirubin, toxins, and other metabolic waste building up, shutting the body down more slowly. With the body's metabolism so out of order, the brainstem, which regulates the body's vital signs, begins to malfunction. Temperature, blood pressure, and pulse may go very high or very low, or fluctuate wildly. Breathing may become irregular and erratic. If the patient seems comfortable, there is no reason to treat these abnormal measurements and signs. Remember, we are treating the patient, not the numbers. As death comes, blood pressure drops, pulse and respirations slow, and finally become undetectable.

Patients in their last days may become unable to wake up and even become unresponsive to pain. Circulation begins to shut down resulting in first cold, pale extremities, then bluish nail beds, followed by the bluish tint extending to fingers, toes, hand and feet, and then arms and legs. The last skin change is "mottling," which is a coarse web pattern of blue on very pale skin, first on the arms and legs and then spreading to the abdomen and chest.

As metabolic changes continue to occur, the brain loses its sensitivity to oxygen levels. The addition of supplemental oxygen (please see chapter 6 on "Shortness of Breath") at this point may only make the patient more aware of their suffering and prolong the painful dying process. Although with low oxygen, one gets a sense of breathlessness, such as when hiking at high altitude, it is not particularly painful. If breathing becomes faster and deeper, it is due to the acid in the blood (CO_2—carbon dioxide—acidifies the blood), which makes the brainstem increase breathing rate and depth to "blow off" the acidic CO_2.

In the last twenty-four to forty-eight hours of life, the large airways may begin to secrete a large amount of thin mucous. This copious thin mucous moves and flutters about with the patient's increased respirations. This fluttering sound is known as the "death rattle." Other than simply an indicator of impending death, it has little if any significance. Although the mucous flutters about in the large airways, the tiny air sacs, where oxygen and CO_2 are transferred, remain clear. Nor is there usually wheezing from constriction of the small to medium airways. If anything, this death rattle indicates good airflow, not bad airflow. However, the noise can be quite distressing to the family at times, especially if they interpret it as increased trouble breathing. The noise is *not* distressing to the patient.

There have been a variety of medications designed to quiet this noise. They are all strongly anticholinergic (AC). These medications include such things as hyoscyamine tablets or atropine eye-drops (given under the tongue). Recent studies have shown none of them to make much difference in the quantity or duration of the secretions. Any hope for improvement of these symptoms would take many hours as these medications only reduce further production of the secretions, not make those that are presently causing the noise suddenly go away. There are also no studies that show that these medications actually provide relief to the patient. It would seem that their primary use is to provide the concerned, caring family with something to do for a symptom bothering them, not the unresponsive patient.

If anything, these anticholinergic medications stand to make the patient *more* uncomfortable with their side effects of constipation, dry mouth, urinary blockage, and delirium with hallucinations and agitation. And certainly, these drugs should *never* be given to patients who have conditions such as COPD/emphysema or congestion from aspiration from trouble swallowing. These secretions are helpful in removing debris from the airways. Drying up these secretions not only impair the removal of foreign material from the lungs, resulting in increased infection risk, but the thickened immobile plugs of mucous caused by these drugs will actually block the airways resulting in lower oxygen levels and increased shortness of breath.

It is the buildup of CO_2, not low levels of oxygen, that causes the most discomfort. Remember what it is like holding your breath under water. It is the CO_2 buildup that makes your body so desperate for air. With dying, this last, and most sensitive drive, gradually lessens. The patient begins to have pauses in their breathing. Breaths begin to come in clusters with increasingly long pauses in between. As CO_2 builds up, the pause ends with a deep breath, followed by breaths that are more and more shallow. The breathing effort gradually weakens and finally breathing stops.

Finally, we wish to discuss our favorite issues indicating that death may be only days away, visitations, and terminal lucidity. Visitations are when you hear or observe the patient pleasantly talking to someone in the room that you cannot see. Often the patient will identify the visitor as a family member or friend who has died in the recent or remote past. These experiences are not associated with delirium, medications, infections, or psychosis. They tend to be comforting and do not cause distress for the patient. In fact, a few days before my mother-in-law died, she frequently would glow with a smile, point out the window, and say, "Look! There's John!". John was her beloved husband who died a few years ago.

As these events are so benign, so common, and not associated with any distress or disease, the American Academy of Hospice and Palliative Medicine (AAHPM) does not consider these visitations pathological or psychotic, nor do they recommend any treatment for them, unless the patient is demonstrating some kind of distress. Remarkably, there have been reported many incidences of family members and caregivers who have reported actually visualizing the same "visitor" that the patient was speaking to. These "third party" visitation experiences, however, *were* met with some (often much) distress. Documentation of these events can be found in the publications of the University of Virginia, Department of Perceptual Studies, such as the books, *The Irreducible Mind* and *Beyond Physicalism*, by Edward F. Kelly, et al.

Another fascinating event that we see, not infrequently, is the phenomenon of *terminal lucidity*. This is when a patient who may be moments from dying, possibly profoundly demented or unconscious for days, suddenly wakes up, speaks perfectly and rationally to the family at the bedside for a few moments, and then closes their eyes and dies.

Visitations and terminal lucidity are consistent with the theory on consciousness (that has had growing scientific support over the past 130 years) that the brain does not produce consciousness but rather filter or limit consciousness. It may be that our consciousness (or soul or spirit) is not an illusion of the neurochemistry in our brains, but rather consciousness is the very real, nonphysical essence of who we are. This has been believed for the past one hundred and fifty thousand years or so. Burial sites of even Neanderthals indicate that they believed that when we die, our spirit leaves the body and goes somewhere else.

The theory states that our brain acts like a television set. The TV allows a single, perfect, invisible broadcast signal to be experienced, often imperfectly, in our sensory world on our TV screen. The brain, similarly, allows the same thing with our consciousness or spirit. But just like a TV receiver is tuned to only one station, in order to block out the overwhelming confusion of broadcasting the one thousand available channels all at once, our brains usually block out all but the small amount of what our consciousness is capable of experiencing. The brain usually only lets through the part of our consciousness required to physically survive on this physical rock we call planet earth. As the brain shuts down during the dying process, interesting things start breaking through, such as visitations and terminal lucidity.

The two books mentioned above are together fourteen hundred pages, much of which is highly technical scientific literature, much of which is so technical that it is essentially inaccessible to the lay public. The extensive parts that are accessible are riveting and potentially life transforming. Even a limited discussion of the mind/brain controversy, and the implications of the current data, especially when it comes to the science/religion debate is far beyond the scope of this book. (But maybe not beyond the scope of our next one, which is in the works!)

Guy with the Cigar

Jennifer was at her wits' end. Her mother, Sophie, who lived in Southern California, had taken a sudden turn for the worse. Sophie had been suffering with Alzheimer's disease for many years. Her dad, Carl, had been caring for her until about three years ago when he suddenly died of a heart attack.

Jennifer had hired live-in care givers to be able to keep Mom in her home. But as Sophie's disease progressed, she began having more difficulty swallowing. Sophie went on to develop pneumonia, becoming bedbound and total care for all her needs. The increased cost for in-home care-givers became more than the family could bear. Jennifer had her mother moved up to her own home in Northern California, to care for her herself. Jennifer's old college roommate and best friend, Connie, who had never met her parents, agreed to give her what help she could.

Jennifer invited Connie over for dinner so she could meet her mom and so they could work out how to share the caregiving duties. Connie parked on the side of the house as usual and used the key under the flower pot to come in through the side garage door. As she hurried into the house, she noticed an elderly gentleman in a plaid shirt with the stub of a cigar in his mouth over by the work-bench in the corner of the garage.

Connie found Jennifer in the kitchen chopping fresh veggies for the salad. Jennifer put down the knife and said, "Thanks so much for coming over. Come on back with me, and I'll introduce you to my mom."

As they walked into Sophie's room, Connie asked, "Who is your friend with the cigar in the garage?"

Jennifer froze. "There shouldn't be anyone in the garage! What did he look like?"

"That's him. Same shirt, same cigar." Connie said, pointing to a photo on Sophie's nightstand.

Jennifer turned white. "That's my dad! You must be mistaken; he died three years ago."

Cautiously they tiptoed back down the hallway, quietly cracked open the door to the garage, and peeked in. They saw no one.

They quickly returned to Sophie's room. But when they checked her, she was no longer breathing, but her usual fretful countenance was replaced with a peaceful smile.

16

FINAL THOUGHTS

There is nothing more terrible than losing someone you love. Yet, in this life everyone must experience such a loss. Western culture treats death as failure of the medical system or as some kind of accident. We always hear, "He lost his battle with…" We spend untold billions of dollars on worthless supplements, risky procedures, and potentially dangerous preventive medications, even in our geriatric population. We view the diagnosis of a terminal illness, even in the very elderly, as "unlucky," as if there were alternatives to dying. The end of life is just as certain and just as natural as its beginning.

We should be viewing life and death with the same expectation as we view the rising and setting of the sun. But because we conceal the natural end of life in hospitals and nursing homes, we are ill prepared to deal with the event, let alone the symptoms, that the end of life brings. For most people, caring for a family member at home, who is expected to die there, is a first-time event. Our goal is to make as many people aware as possible of the help, support, and preparation that our caring hospice teams can bring to families.

In this time of pain, we are deeply grateful that we can share with you perspectives and advice that you may not find elsewhere in the medical community. We have acquired many years of experience, dealing with those who are completing their pilgrimage among us. Never forget that grieving is the risk and cost of loving. The greater the love you have felt for someone, the greater the grief at their loss. The grief you are feeling is simply the shadow cast by the love you have had the privilege of sharing with your loved one. We, and the hospice team that you hopefully have chosen, are profoundly honored and humbled that you would allow us be a part of this very sacred time for your family.

The pain of knowing that you are soon to lose a loved one is often compounded by fear of the unknown regarding the journey on which you are embarking. Losing your loved one can be so difficult, and their suffering, as well as yours, can be great. Apprehension and doubt are normal when you feel you are facing it alone and do not know what to expect. This is why hospice exists, and also why this book exists. We have been there thousands of times. The hospice team faces the darkness of death daily, and we know we have the tools to minimize the suffering and pain. We just need the opportunity and the time to provide the help needed. The earlier we can enroll an eligible patient in hospice, the sooner and more assuredly we can help bring comfort and peace.

At a time that seems so dark, it is hard to believe there is hope of any kind. Many are wary as false hope may have been offered in the past. In hospice we strive never to make false promises or set unrealistic goals. We seek to build bridges of trust with families, sometimes in only a very short period of time. Only then can the realistic hope of a comfortable and peaceful transition from this life be achieved through a dignified departure.

We did not make up the stories we added at the ends of the chapters. They are either from our first-hand experiences or the events related to us by reliable hospice staff and reluctant families. Those who told us of these events were not looking for notoriety. In fact, most of them did not want to be identified. Most often they would say something like, "I don't want people to think I'm crazy, but..." Most people who have experienced these types of difficult-to-explain phenomena are very private about them. These are moments they treasure as a special gift from their departed loved one. We are fascinated by these stories because of how little we know about what happens after we die.

Perhaps the best glimpse we have "behind the curtain" involves near-death experiences, or NDEs. These were often dismissed as rare, fanciful anecdotes, but they are now being seriously studied. The Department of Perceptual Studies at the University of Virginia, School of Medicine, has looked at over twenty-five hundred such cases. It is not our intention to make any religious claims. Our only intention is to report what this data has shown, that it is highly probable that our consciousness (soul or spirit) survives the death of the body.

NDEs occur when people are revived after being clinically dead (no heartbeat or respirations, no chemical or electrical brain activity). Although accounts vary greatly, there are general themes to these experiences. "My whole life flashed before my eyes." "I was in a tunnel [cultural variations substitute 'cave', 'tube', or 'pipe'] moving toward a bright light." There is usually the perception of floating above their bodies and looking down on the frantic resuscitation attempts. These experiences are generally associated with overwhelming feelings of love and peace, as well as a profound reluctance to return to their bodies.

What makes these stories remarkable and believable is that these survivors could see things out of their bodies that they would not be able to see with their physical eyes. For example, details of labels on the tops of operating room lamps, unusual and detailed behaviors of hospital staff (even though their faces were covered with drapes), activities of family members in other locations of the hospital (including the name of the show on the TV playing in the corner).

With their brain activity completely shut down, they appear to have *enhanced* perceptions and vivid memories (persistent, detailed recollection of these events even decades after they occurred). They have profound, life-changing spiritual experiences (returning more compassionate, less materialistic, and no fear of dying again). Many describe the feeling of connection to a universal consciousness characterized by unconditional love. Other experiences include distortion of time or the absence of the passage of time. Yet another feeling is having access to all knowledge and all events everywhere in the universe.

Much of the scientific community deny that these phenomena exist, as most feel that consciousness is what the brain *does*. But these NDEs and hospice experiences do indeed exist. Similar stories, like the ones at the ends of our chapters, are experienced on a daily basis in the hospice community. When reality does not behave according to our theories, we must look at alternatives to our theories. What if the brain is not what *produces* our consciousness, but rather is the organ that *attaches our consciousness* to one specific body?

It is beginning to appear that when the brain is very stressed or shutting down, our consciousness starts to lose some of its connections to our brain and body. By doing so, it may have access to information and awareness that it did not have before. Imagine being in a windowless room. The sun can only get in through holes or cracks in the roof. Through these enlarging "cracks in the roof," we may get things like NDEs, visitations, and terminal lucidity. This new theory of the mind suggests that previously unexplainable mental phenomena may be better understood if the brain is not what produces the mind through its chemical and electrical activity but rather filters or blocks experiences and information usually beyond its reach. Things like genius, creativity, talent, savant abilities to do otherwise impossible mental mathematics, lifetime perfect (photographic) memory, psychic abilities, and intuition may be things from "out there" that some brains fail to block or filter out.

How could our consciousness have such freedom and access to all that information? The view we have from our bodies is like the view we have driving a car from San Francisco to New York. We can see a short distance in front, behind, to the right, and to the left. The view we have when we are not limited by the constraints of our bodies is like the view from the Google Earth satellite. We can see the entire hemisphere all at once or focus down on any pinpoint of turf, anywhere, for as long as we like. Right now, the view of the entire hemisphere is not available to us.

The tiny glimpse we get from these spiritual experiences may point to confirmations of the truths taught for millennia by the great faiths. Perhaps, indeed, in the search for the meaning of life, we should focus on the centrality of love and relationship, the equality and unity of all human beings, and finally, that we may actually have an eternity to live with the choices that we make in this life. All I can guarantee you is that we will all find out.

It has been an honor and privilege for us to try to bring peace, comfort, and dignity to those souls who are leaving this world. They may be entering into a new existence, even more amazing than what they found when they entered this world. May this book bring you hope and comfort and continue the work that we have done in person for so much of our professional lives. And for this opportunity, we give you our profound thanks.

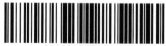
35200669R00078

Made in the USA
San Bernardino, CA
08 May 2019